The Caregiver

In

Internal Medicine

The complete Guide

MARTIN STERLING

Table of contents

Chapter 1: Introduction to Internal Medicine   11

- Understanding Internal Medicine:
  definition and scope   12

- The orderly: a pillar of the Internal
  Medicine department   15

- Common pathologies in internal medicine   18

- A holistic approach to the patient   22

Chapter 2: The caregiver's essential skills   27

- Basic medical knowledge   28

- Specific care techniques in internal
  medicine   32

- Effective communication with the
  multidisciplinary team   37

- Management of medical tools and
  equipment   41

Chapter 3: Daily care in internal medicine   49

- Monitoring vital signs and clinical
  parameters   50

- Assistance with nursing procedures   55

- Pain management and patient comfort   60

- Prevention of pressure sores and nosocomial infections   66

Chapter 4: Helping the patient   73

- Establishing therapeutic communication   74

- Psychological support and guidance   80

- Respect for patient dignity and privacy   85

- Managing difficult or end-of-life patients   91

Chapter 5: Emergency management   97

- Recognizing clinical warning signs   98

- Emergency protocols and internal procedures   102

- The caregiver's role in critical interventions   109

- Stress management in emergency situations   114

Chapter 6: Ethics and professional conduct   121

- Confidentiality and medical secrecy   122

- Patient rights and informed consent   127

- Professional practices and legal responsibilities   133

- Compliance with safety protocols and standards   140

Chapter 7: Challenges facing the Internal Medicine Department   147

- Workload and time management   148

- Adapting to technological and medical developments   153

- Occupational risk prevention   160

- Work-life balance   164

Chapter 8: Innovative technologies in internal medicine   171

- The impact of telemedicine on the role of the caregiver   172

- Using digital tools to monitor patients   175

- Training in new medical technologies   180

- Security and confidentiality of patient data   186

Chapter 9: Case studies and practical examples   193

- Analysis of complex clinical situations   194

- Handling contingencies and emergencies   200

- Problem-solving strategies   206

- Feedback and lessons learned   212

Chapter 10: Conclusion

Chapter 10: Conclusion   219

- The impact of the orderly in Internal Medicine   220

- Incentives for future professionals   223

- The future of the nursing profession   226

- Useful resources and references   229

« *Internal Medicine is the heart of the hospital, where the complexity of disease meets the compassion of the caregivers. The caregiver plays an essential role, combining technical know-how and humanity to accompany each patient on the road to recovery.* »

Chapter 1

Introduction to Internal Medicine

- Understanding Internal Medicine: definition and scope

Internal Medicine is a fundamental medical specialty dedicated to the comprehensive care of adult patients with complex, often multisystem pathologies. It is positioned at the crossroads of many medical disciplines, offering a holistic approach that considers the individual as a whole, rather than focusing on a specific organ or system. The discipline demands extensive medical knowledge, in-depth analytical skills and the versatility to manage varied and often interconnected clinical situations.

Definition of Internal Medicine

Internal Medicine is the specialty dedicated to the diagnosis, treatment and prevention of adult diseases, particularly those affecting several organ systems. It encompasses a broad spectrum of pathologies, from acute conditions to complex chronic diseases. Internists are often called upon for their expertise in cases where the diagnosis is uncertain, where several conditions coexist, or when medical complications arise in patients hospitalized for other reasons.

This specialty focuses on an in-depth understanding of the pathophysiological mechanisms of disease, enabling a rational, personalized approach to patient care. Internists play a key role in coordinating care, collaborating with other specialists to ensure integrated, coherent management.

Scope and importance of internal medicine

The scope of Internal Medicine is vast, covering many subspecialties such as endocrinology, gastroenterology, pneumology, nephrology, hematology, infectiology, rheumatology and many others. This interdisciplinarity enables internists to manage complex clinical situations, where several pathologies may interact or mask each other.

In the hospital setting, the Internal Medicine department is often the point of referral for patients with non-specific symptoms, rare diseases or unexplained syndromes. Patients admitted to this department may suffer from autoimmune diseases, systemic infections, metabolic disorders, hematological cancers or multivisceral failures. The ability to integrate clinical, biological and imaging information is essential to establishing an accurate diagnosis and devising an effective treatment plan.

The role of the nursing auxiliary in internal medicine

In this complex context, the nursing auxiliary plays a crucial role in the care team. Their contribution is not limited to basic care, but extends to active participation in clinical monitoring, prevention of complications and psychological support for patients. In Internal Medicine, where health conditions can evolve rapidly, the orderly is often the first to detect subtle changes in the patient's condition, thanks to continuous, attentive observation.

The complexity of the pathologies encountered requires the caregiver to have a sound knowledge of the clinical signs associated with different illnesses. For example, recognizing the early signs of cardiac decompensation, respiratory failure or severe infection can enable rapid intervention by the medical team. In addition, caregivers need to be familiar with the specific protocols associated with complex treatments, such as infusions of immunosuppressive drugs, care of immunocompromised patients or management of invasive medical devices.

Holistic Patient Approach

The holistic approach is at the heart of Internal Medicine practice. Each patient is considered as a whole, with attention paid not only to their physical symptoms, but also to their psychological, social and environmental state. Patients with chronic or complex illnesses may experience anxiety, depression or distress related to their condition. The caregiver plays a key role in identifying these non-medical needs and putting in place appropriate support measures.

For example, a patient with type 2 diabetes with renal and cardiovascular complications may also suffer from social isolation or economic difficulties that impact on their health. The caregiver, in collaboration with the multidisciplinary team, can help refer the patient to social assistance services, therapeutic education programs or support groups.

Interaction with the Multidisciplinary Team

Internal medicine requires close collaboration between various healthcare professionals. The nursing auxiliary is an essential link in this chain, ensuring continuity of care and efficient transmission of information. They collaborate with doctors, nurses, physiotherapists, dieticians, psychologists and social workers to draw up and implement the patient's care plan.

Communication is a fundamental aspect of this collaboration. The caregiver must master medical language to understand instructions, report observations accurately and participate actively in team meetings. For example, reporting a change in diuresis, the appearance of edema, or changes in the patient's state of consciousness can be crucial to medical management.

Challenges and Opportunities in Internal Medicine

Working in Internal Medicine presents unique challenges for the orderly. The diversity of pathologies, the complexity of cases and the emotional burden associated with caring for critically ill patients can be demanding. However, it also offers opportunities for learning and professional development. Caregivers gain rich and varied experience, strengthen their clinical skills and develop resilience in the face of difficult situations.

In addition, the internal medicine caregiver can play a role in patient education, providing information on daily care, symptom management and treatment adherence. This educational dimension is essential to promote patient autonomy and improve long-term outcomes.

- The orderly: a pillar of the Internal Medicine department

At the heart of the Internal Medicine department, the orderly occupies a central position, playing an indispensable role in the day-to-day running and quality of patient care. His or her contribution goes far beyond technical tasks, encompassing an essential human dimension that makes him or her an essential pillar of the care team.

An essential presence for patients

The nursing auxiliary is often the patient's first contact with healthcare personnel. Through their empathetic approach and availability, they create a bond of trust that facilitates overall care. In Internal Medicine, where patients often present complex pathologies and fluctuating states of health, this privileged relationship enables us to better understand individual needs and adapt care accordingly.

Their constant presence at patients' bedsides enables them to detect subtle changes in their state of health at an early stage. Whether it's an alteration in consciousness, the appearance of new symptoms or a change in vital signs, the caregiver is in the front line to observe and report these developments to the nursing and medical team. This vigilance helps to prevent complications and to intervene early in the event of an emergency.

Versatile technical expertise

The diversity of pathologies in internal medicine requires the nursing auxiliary to have solid training and great versatility. They master basic care tasks such as personal hygiene, feeding and mobilization of patients, while being proficient in the use of specific medical devices. They participate in clinical monitoring, taking measurements such as temperature, blood pressure and blood sugar, and ensuring that monitoring equipment is working properly.

Their role also involves in-depth knowledge of hygiene protocols to prevent nosocomial infections, which are particularly crucial in the case of immunocompromised patients or those with invasive devices. By rigorously applying these protocols, the orderly contributes to patient safety and quality of care.

A communication link within the multidisciplinary team

The caregiver plays a key role in transmitting information between the patient, the family and the nursing team. They ensure smooth, efficient communication, accurately reporting their observations and the needs expressed by the patient. This is essential for continuity of care and coordination between different healthcare professionals.

By taking part in team meetings and communications, the caregiver brings a valuable perspective based on his or her proximity to the patient. They work closely with nurses, doctors, physiotherapists, dieticians and social workers, helping to draw up and implement personalized care plans.

Psychological and human support

Beyond the technical aspects, the caregiver offers indispensable psychological support to patients who are often confronted with anxiety-provoking situations, pain or uncertainty linked to their state of health. By listening attentively, showing kindness and empathy, they help patients to express their feelings, overcome their fears and maintain positive morale.

This human dimension is particularly important in internal medicine, where chronic or serious illness can cause significant emotional distress. The caregiver accompanies the patient throughout his or her course of treatment, creating a reassuring environment conducive to recovery.

Commitment to ongoing training and professional development

Aware of the constant evolution of medical practices, nursing assistants are committed to continuous training to keep their knowledge and skills up to date. Participation in specialized training courses, practical workshops and professional development programs helps to improve the quality of care and meet new departmental requirements.

In internal medicine, ongoing training is essential to mastering new technologies, understanding therapeutic advances and adapting to innovative protocols. In this way, caregivers strengthen their ability to provide safe, appropriate care, while enhancing their role within the healthcare team.

Managing complex situations and emergencies

The Internal Medicine department is often faced with unexpected situations or medical emergencies. The orderly must be able to react quickly, applying the appropriate procedures and alerting the medical team. Their knowledge of emergency protocols and their ability to remain calm and act effectively are crucial to patient safety.

He also plays an active role in managing complex situations, such as patients with multiple co-morbidities or cognitive disorders. His adaptability and flexibility enable him to offer personalized care despite the challenges inherent in these situations.

Respect for professional ethics and deontology

The nursing auxiliary practises its profession in strict compliance with ethical and deontological principles. They ensure the confidentiality of medical information, respect patients' rights and preserve their dignity and privacy. In internal medicine, where patients can be particularly vulnerable, this ethical vigilance is fundamental.

It is also attentive to issues of informed consent, ensuring that patients understand the care they are receiving and respecting their choices and wishes. This approach builds trust between the patient and the care team, fostering respectful, humane care.

A key player in promoting quality of care

Through their day-to-day commitment, orderlies actively contribute to the continuous improvement of care quality in Internal Medicine. They take part in quality initiatives, internal audits and the evaluation of professional practices. Their feedback and suggestions can lead to improvements in the department's care protocols and procedures.

Working with the team, he or she supports the implementation of innovative projects designed to optimize patient care, improve comfort and reduce the risks associated with care.

• Common pathologies in internal medicine
Internal Medicine is a vast and complex specialty, encompassing a multitude of pathologies affecting various body systems. It is mainly aimed at adults with non-surgical medical conditions that are often polymorphous and interconnected. For caregivers, understanding these pathologies is essential in order to adapt their care, monitor patients effectively and collaborate closely with the nursing team.

Cardiovascular diseases

Cardiovascular disorders are common in internal medicine. Among them, heart failure, characterized by the heart's inability to ensure sufficient blood flow, requires rigorous monitoring of clinical signs such as edema of the lower limbs, dyspnea, fatigue and orthopnea. The caregiver must be attentive to weight variations, a sign of hydrosodic retention, and ensure water restriction if prescribed.

Hypertension, often asymptomatic, can lead to serious complications such as stroke or myocardial infarction. Regular measurement of blood pressure and observation of symptoms such as headaches, dizziness or visual disturbances are essential.

Metabolic and Endocrine Diseases

Diabetes mellitus, particularly type 2 diabetes, is a common pathology requiring special attention. The caregiver must master the capillary blood glucose technique, and recognize the signs of hypoglycemia (sweating, trembling, confusion) and hyperglycemia (intense thirst, polyuria, fatigue). They must also help educate patients about healthy eating and the importance of adherence to treatment.

Thyroid disorders, such as hypothyroidism and hyperthyroidism, present a variety of clinical pictures. The caregiver must be alert to signs such as bradycardia, chilliness and weight gain in hypothyroidism, or tachycardia, weight loss and excitability in hyperthyroidism.

Infectious Diseases

Infections are at the heart of Internal Medicine, whether community-acquired or nosocomial. Infectious pneumopathies, for example, require monitoring of respiratory rate, oxygen saturation, body temperature and sputum appearance. Caregivers must rigorously apply hygiene measures to prevent cross-transmission, including hand-washing and wearing personal protective equipment.

Sepsis and opportunistic infections in immunocompromised patients (such as those with HIV or on immunosuppressive drugs) require extra vigilance. Signs of infection may be discreet, and the caregiver must be alert to any change in general condition, such as unexplained fever, chills or altered consciousness.

Respiratory diseases

Chronic obstructive pulmonary disease (COPD), including chronic bronchitis and emphysema, is common. The caregiver must monitor signs of respiratory distress, the use of accessory respiratory muscles, cyanosis and the patient's ability to expectorate effectively. He/she helps set up oxygen therapy at the prescribed flow rates, and monitors the risk of hypercapnia in at-risk patients.

Asthma, although often managed on an outpatient basis, may require hospitalization for severe exacerbations. Caregivers must be able to recognize the signs of an acute asthma attack and quickly assist the medical team.

Rheumatological and autoimmune diseases

Pathologies such as rheumatoid arthritis, systemic lupus erythematosus and scleroderma are complex, affecting several systems. Patients may present with joint pain, skin, kidney or lung damage. The caregiver must assess pain, help with mobilization to prevent ankylosis, and monitor for signs of systemic damage.

The immunosuppressive treatments used in these diseases increase the risk of infection, requiring close monitoring and strict preventive measures.

Hematological diseases

Anemia, leukemia and coagulation disorders are commonly treated in internal medicine. Caregivers must be alert to signs of anemia (pallor, fatigue, tachycardia), hemorrhagic signs (petechiae, ecchymosis, mucous membrane bleeding) and signs of infection in neutropenic patients.

Handling labile blood products for transfusion requires knowledge of blood compatibility protocols, verification procedures and monitoring of transfusion reactions.

Gastrointestinal and liver diseases

Viral hepatitis, liver cirrhosis and chronic inflammatory bowel disease (IBD) such as Crohn's disease or ulcerative colitis are common. The caregiver must watch for signs of digestive bleeding, jaundice, ascites and deteriorating nutritional status.

Nutritional management is often a key element, requiring collaboration with the dietician. The caregiver is involved in monitoring food intake, assisting with feeding if necessary, and measuring intake and output to assess fluid balance.

Kidney Diseases

Acute or chronic renal failure requires strict monitoring of diuresis, blood pressure, weight and signs of edema. The caregiver must be familiar with the principles of water and sodium restriction, and understand the importance of monitoring electrolytes, particularly potassium, variations in which can have serious cardiac consequences.

For dialysis patients, caregivers must be familiar with the specific care required for vascular access, such as arteriovenous fistula, and monitor for signs of infection or malfunction.

Neurological diseases

Although some neurological diseases are the responsibility of specialized neurology, Internal Medicine also deals with conditions such as stroke, metabolic encephalopathy and peripheral neuropathy. Caregivers must monitor the patient's state of consciousness, motor and sensory functions, and help prevent complications linked to immobility, such as bedsores or deep vein thrombosis.

Communicating with aphasic or cognitively impaired patients requires special skills in terms of patience, understanding and adapting communication methods.

Oncological pathologies

Internal medicine is often involved in the care of patients with hematological cancers or solid tumors in the systemic phase. Treatments such as chemotherapy have significant side-effects that the caregiver needs to be aware of: nausea, vomiting, mucositis, bone marrow aplasia. Monitoring vital parameters, preventing infections and providing nutritional support are essential.

Associated psychiatric disorders

Internal medicine patients may present with concomitant psychiatric disorders, such as depression, anxiety or confusional states. The caregiver must be able to recognize these signs, adopt a reassuring attitude and report any changes in behavior to the medical team.

Polypathology and geriatrics

Elderly patients account for a significant proportion of hospital admissions in Internal Medicine, often with complex polypathologies. Caregivers must be alert to the risk of falls, malnutrition, dehydration and cognitive disorders such as delirium. Comprehensive care requires a multidisciplinary approach, with care adapted to the patient's abilities.

- A holistic approach to the patient

In the context of Internal Medicine, the holistic approach to the patient is of paramount importance. It involves considering the individual as a whole, taking into account not only his or her physical symptoms, but also his or her psychological, social, cultural and spiritual dimensions. This integrative vision recognizes that every aspect of a patient's life can influence his or her state of health and healing process. For the caregiver, adopting a holistic approach means providing personalized care that addresses the complex and unique needs of each patient.

Understanding the whole patient

The holistic approach begins with a thorough understanding of the patient as a whole human being. This means knowing their personal history, medical history, living conditions, beliefs, values and social relationships. For example, a patient suffering from a chronic illness such as diabetes may also experience anxiety related to their condition, financial difficulties in accessing care, or a lack of family support. Caregivers need to be aware of these factors to adapt their care appropriately.

The importance of empathic communication

Open, empathetic communication is essential to establishing a relationship of trust with the patient. The caregiver must practice active listening, paying attention to the patient's verbal and non-verbal concerns. This means paying attention to body language, tone of voice and facial expressions. Effective communication helps to better understand the patient's needs, reduce anxiety and actively involve them in their own care process.

Taking psychological dimensions into account

The patient's emotions and mental state play a crucial role in his or her recovery. Stress, depression and anxiety can weaken the immune system and aggravate physical symptoms. The caregiver must be able to recognize signs of emotional distress and provide appropriate support. This can include reassuring words, providing a calm and secure environment, or coordinating with specialized professionals such as psychologists.

Social and cultural considerations

Social factors, such as family support, friendships and living conditions, also influence patient health. Similarly, cultural and religious beliefs can affect the perception of illness and the way the patient reacts to treatment. Caregivers must respect these aspects and adapt their care accordingly. For example, it may be necessary to take cultural food preferences into account when planning meals, or to respect certain religious practices.

Promoting patient autonomy

Encouraging patients to actively participate in their own care is a key component of the holistic approach. The caregiver must provide clear, comprehensible information about the disease and treatment, enabling the patient to make informed decisions. By promoting autonomy, the patient's self-confidence is strengthened and adherence to treatment is improved. This can take the form of learning self-care techniques or participating in the development of the care plan.

Interprofessional collaboration

The holistic approach requires close collaboration between all members of the care team. Caregivers play a central role, coordinating their actions with those of nurses, doctors, physiotherapists, dieticians and social workers. This synergy ensures that all aspects of the patient's needs are covered. For example, if a patient has difficulty moving around, the caregiver can work with the physiotherapist to set up suitable exercises.

Pain and comfort management

Pain is a subjective experience that affects the patient's physical and mental well-being. The caregiver must regularly assess the level of pain using appropriate scales, and report any increase to the medical team. In addition, they may apply non-pharmacological methods to relieve pain, such as repositioning, massage or relaxation. Ensuring the patient's comfort also includes looking after hygiene, keeping the environment clean and preventing bedsores.

Emotional and spiritual support

Emotional support is essential, especially for patients facing serious or chronic illnesses. The caregiver must demonstrate empathy, offer a comforting presence and be available to listen to the patient's concerns. Some patients may also have spiritual needs, whether religious or linked to existential issues. Respecting these needs may involve facilitating access to a chaplain or creating a space for meditation or prayer.

Prevention and health education

The holistic approach includes health promotion and disease prevention. The caregiver can play an educational role by informing the patient about preventive measures, healthy lifestyle habits and the management of his or her medical condition. For example, he or she can explain the importance of a balanced diet, regular exercise or compliance with medication. Health education empowers patients and helps improve long-term outcomes.

Adapting to change and transition

Internal medicine patients can undergo major transitions, such as the transition from hospital to home, or adapting to a new reality of living with a chronic illness. The caregiver must support the patient through these phases, facilitating discharge planning, coordinating home services or referring to community resources. This continuity of care is essential to maintaining the patient's well-being after hospitalization.

Respect for ethics and confidentiality

The holistic approach respects the ethical principles of the profession. Caregivers must guarantee the confidentiality of patient information, obtain informed consent for care and respect patients' decisions, even when they choose to refuse treatment. Treating patients with dignity and respect is fundamental, regardless of their lifestyle choices, culture or state of health.

Continuous professional development

To provide high-quality, holistic care, caregivers must engage in ongoing training. This includes updating medical knowledge, perfecting communication skills and raising awareness of different cultures and practices. Professional development enables the caregiver to adapt to developments in medicine and the changing needs of patients.

Chapter 2

The caregiver's essential skills

- Basic medical knowledge

In the demanding field of internal medicine, mastery of basic medical knowledge is a fundamental pillar for the nursing auxiliary. This skill is not simply an accumulation of theoretical knowledge, but the foundation on which effective care, patient safety and harmonious collaboration with the multidisciplinary team are built. Understanding the essential principles of anatomy, physiology, common pathologies and treatments enables the nursing auxiliary to act with discernment and responsiveness in an often complex clinical environment.

The importance of understanding anatomy and physiology

A sound knowledge of human anatomy and physiology is essential for understanding the body's normal functioning and recognizing signs of dysfunction. This includes understanding the cardiovascular, respiratory, digestive, nervous, endocrine, urinary and musculoskeletal systems. For example, knowing how the heart pumps blood and how the lungs exchange gases helps the caregiver interpret vital signs and detect abnormalities such as tachycardia, hypertension or dyspnea.

This in-depth understanding also enables us to anticipate patients' needs. A patient suffering from renal failure will require particular attention to water and electrolyte balance. Knowledge of renal functions helps the caregiver to monitor diuresis, recognize signs of edema or hyperkalemia, and follow specific dietary recommendations.

Knowledge of common pathologies in internal medicine

Internal medicine covers a wide range of complex diseases. Familiarity with common pathologies enables the caregiver to understand the issues involved in management, and to adapt interventions accordingly. For example, understanding the mechanisms of diabetes mellitus helps to grasp the importance of glycemic monitoring, diet management and recognizing the signs of hypoglycemia or hyperglycemia.

Similarly, knowing the characteristics of heart failure, such as reduced cardiac output and fluid retention, enables the caregiver to monitor the patient's daily weight, assess edema of the lower limbs and report any abnormal shortness of breath. This vigilance helps prevent acute decompensation and optimize treatment.

Understanding treatments and therapeutic protocols

Internal medicine patients often receive complex treatments, including a variety of medications, intravenous infusions, immunosuppressive therapies or anticoagulants. Caregivers need to understand the general principles of these treatments to ensure appropriate monitoring and prevent complications.

For example, knowing the potential side effects of antibiotics enables you to monitor for the appearance of allergic reactions, digestive disorders or fungal superinfections. Similarly, understanding how oral anticoagulants work helps you to be alert to signs of bleeding, such as spontaneous bruising, gum bleeding or hematuria.

Mastery of therapeutic protocols also includes knowledge of procedures for administering treatments, such as preparing infusions, complying with asepsis rules when caring for central venous catheters or managing infusion pumps. Caregivers must be able to check flow rates, recognize equipment alarms and report any anomalies.

Clinical monitoring and interpretation of vital signs

Regularly taking vital signs is an essential task, requiring not only precise technique, but also the ability to interpret them. Understanding the clinical implications of variations in temperature, pulse, blood pressure, respiratory rate and oxygen saturation enables the caregiver to detect signs of deterioration at an early stage.

For example, tachycardia associated with hypotension may indicate incipient shock, requiring immediate medical intervention. A high fever in a neutropenic patient is an infectious emergency that must be reported without delay. The caregiver must therefore be able to relate these data to the patient's clinical condition and act accordingly.

Knowledge of hygiene and infection prevention measures

Preventing nosocomial infections is a major challenge in the hospital environment. Mastery of hospital hygiene skills is essential for nursing auxiliaries. This includes hand-washing techniques, proper use of personal protective equipment, medical waste management and compliance with standard and additional precautions.

Understanding the modes of transmission of infectious agents enables caregivers to apply appropriate preventive measures. For example, knowing that certain bacteria are transmitted by direct contact encourages the reinforcement of isolation measures for patients who are carriers. Similarly, knowledge of the risks associated with invasive devices, such as urinary catheters or venous catheters, guides care to prevent associated infections.

Raising awareness of ethical and legal principles

The practice of nursing care is governed by ethical principles and legal obligations. Knowledge of patients' rights, respect for their dignity and privacy, and confidentiality of medical information are essential. Understanding the notions of informed consent, professional secrecy and legal responsibility protects both patient and professional.

For example, caregivers must be aware that they cannot divulge any information about a patient's state of health without the patient's consent. They must also be aware of the limits of their field of competence, and avoid performing acts reserved for nurses or doctors.

Constant updating of knowledge

Medicine is a constantly evolving field. New pathologies emerge, care protocols are regularly updated, and technological advances modify practices. Caregivers must engage in ongoing training to keep their knowledge and skills up to date.

This can take the form of attending in-house training courses, seminars, reading professional publications or exchanging ideas with colleagues. For example, the emergence of new antibiotic-resistant infectious strains means that hygiene and treatment measures need to be adapted, and caregivers need to be familiar with these if they are to be effective.

Integrating knowledge into daily practice

Mastery of basic medical knowledge is only fully effective if it is integrated into daily practice. Caregivers must be able to mobilize their knowledge proactively, anticipating patients' needs, adapting their care and taking an active part in overall care.

For example, by knowing the risks of thrombosis in a bedridden patient, the caregiver can encourage early mobilization, apply compression stockings if prescribed, and be alert to signs of pain or swelling in the lower limbs. This practical application of knowledge enhances the quality of care and patient safety.

Collaboration with the care team thanks to shared knowledge

A good understanding of medical concepts facilitates communication with other members of the care team. The caregiver can use appropriate technical language to convey observations, understand medical guidelines and participate in clinical discussions.

For example, reporting a patient with decreased diuresis associated with peripheral oedema and high blood pressure enables the medical team to react quickly to adjust treatment. This effective collaboration is based on a shared medical knowledge base.

- Specific care techniques in internal medicine

Internal Medicine is a specialty rich in pathological diversity, requiring specific care techniques adapted to the complex needs of patients. The nursing auxiliary plays a crucial role here, applying precise technical skills to contribute to the effective overall management of patients. This chapter explores the main specific care techniques in Internal Medicine, highlighting the importance of precision, rigor and adaptation to different clinical situations.

Drug administration and monitoring

Medication administration is an essential part of internal medicine care. Although the act of dispensing medication is often reserved for the nurse, the orderly plays an active role in patient preparation and post-administration monitoring.

- **Preparing the patient:** The caregiver ensures that the patient is ready to take the medication, by checking his or her identity, making sure he or she is comfortable and explaining the procedure if necessary. For example, for a patient requiring an intravenous infusion, the caregiver prepares the equipment, ensures hygiene of the insertion site and supports the patient during the procedure.

- **Post-administration monitoring:** After taking the medication, the caregiver observes the patient for any undesirable effects. They monitor vital signs, note skin reactions, assess pain and immediately report any abnormalities to the nurse or doctor.

- **Management of administration devices:** The orderly is responsible for the maintenance and proper operation of devices such as infusion pumps, peripheral venous catheters and gastric tubes. They ensure that lines are patent, change tubing in accordance with protocols and prevent infections by observing asepsis rules.

In-depth clinical monitoring techniques

Clinical monitoring is at the heart of the nursing auxiliary's role in internal medicine. It requires constant attention and precise knowledge of assessment techniques.

- **Measurement of advanced vital parameters:** In addition to taking temperature, pulse and blood pressure, the nursing auxiliary may be required to measure oxygen saturation with a saturometer, assess respiratory frequency and perform capillary blood sugar tests on diabetic patients.

- **Pain assessment:** Using appropriate scales (such as the numerical or visual analog scale), the caregiver quantifies the patient's pain, which is essential for adjusting analgesic treatments and improving comfort.

- **Observation of clinical signs:** Caregivers are trained to recognize signs of deterioration such as cyanosis, edema, pallor, altered consciousness or abnormalities in urine and stools. These observations are crucial to rapid intervention.

Care specific to chronic pathologies

Patients with chronic illnesses require tailored care to manage their condition and prevent complications.

- **Diabetes:** The nursing auxiliary takes part in glycemic monitoring, and helps with therapeutic education by explaining the importance of a balanced diet, physical activity and compliance with treatment. They also monitor the patient's feet for ulcerative lesions.

- **Heart failure:** Monitoring daily weight, diuresis, signs of edema and dyspnea is essential. The caregiver encourages the patient to adopt hygienic-dietary measures, such as limiting salt intake.

- **Chronic respiratory diseases:** For patients with COPD or asthma, the caregiver ensures the correct application of inhalation devices, encourages breathing exercises and monitors for signs of respiratory distress.

Hygiene and infection prevention techniques

Infection prevention is a priority in internal medicine, particularly in immunocompromised patients.

- **Rigorous asepsis:** During care, the caregiver applies asepsis techniques, uses sterile equipment and follows protocols for dressings, catheters and drains.

- **Hand hygiene:** Hand washing is the most effective measure for preventing the transmission of infectious agents. Caregivers follow the five WHO guidelines for hand hygiene.

- **Standard and additional precautions:** He follows standard precautions for all patients and applies additional precautions (contact, droplets, air) according to pathologies, using appropriate personal protective equipment.

Mobilization and prevention of complications related to immobility

Prolonged immobility can lead to severe complications, such as pressure sores, deep vein thrombosis and muscle wasting.

- **Early mobilization:** The caregiver encourages and helps the patient to mobilize as soon as possible, in collaboration with the physiotherapist. This may include simple bed exercises, assistance with getting up and walking.

- **Pressure sore prevention:** Regular changes of position, use of suitable supports (pressure sore mattresses, cushions) and monitoring of skin integrity, particularly at pressure points.

- **Muscle stimulation:** The caregiver can guide the patient through active or passive exercises to maintain muscle tone and prevent atrophy.

Palliative care management and end-of-life support

In internal medicine, the nursing auxiliary is often confronted with palliative or end-of-life patients.

- **Symptom relief:** Participates in the implementation of measures to relieve pain, dyspnea, anxiety and other uncomfortable symptoms, following established protocols.

- **Emotional support:** The caregiver offers a comforting presence, listens to the concerns of the patient and family, and promotes a peaceful environment.

- **Respecting the patient's wishes:** In collaboration with the nursing team, he/she ensures that the patient's wishes concerning his/her care, comfort and dignity are respected.

Therapeutic communication techniques

Communication is an essential tool for the caregiver, both to gather information and to provide reassurance.

- **Active listening:** By paying full attention to the patient, the caregiver better understands his or her needs and concerns, enabling personalized care.

- **Appropriate language:** Using clear language, avoiding medical jargon and ensuring that the patient understands the information given is crucial to effective communication.

- **Non-verbal communication:** Gestures, eye contact, facial expressions and tone of voice are all ways of establishing a relationship of trust with the patient.

Use of medical technologies

Technological advances have introduced new tools into daily practice.

- **Vital signs monitors:** The caregiver must be proficient in the use of multiparametric monitors, understand alarms and interpret data for continuous monitoring.

- **Infusion pumps and electric syringes:** Monitor equipment, check settings, change consumables and report any malfunctions.

- **Digital tools:** Entering data into computerized patient records requires expertise in healthcare software, to guarantee traceability and confidentiality of information.

Specific techniques for different clinical situations

- **Care of infectious patients:** The orderly follows isolation protocols, manages infectious waste, and takes care to limit the spread of pathogens.

- **Acute pain management:** applies non-pharmacological techniques such as relaxation, distraction or repositioning to relieve pain.

- **Management of swallowing disorders:** In dysphagic patients, the caregiver adapts the texture of food, supervises feeding and prevents the risk of a false start.

Training and adaptation of techniques

Care techniques evolve with medical progress and the specific needs of patients.

- **Ongoing training:** The nursing auxiliary regularly attends training courses to keep abreast of new practices and protocols.

- **Adaptability:** When faced with new situations or rare pathologies, he/she is flexible, seeks information from the team and adapts his/her techniques accordingly.

- **Sharing knowledge:** By collaborating with colleagues, the orderly contributes to improving practices and harmonizing care within the department.

- Effective communication with the multidisciplinary team
In the complex world of internal medicine, effective communication within the multidisciplinary team is an essential component of quality patient care. The nursing auxiliary occupies a central position in this system, often acting as the direct link between the patient and other healthcare professionals. Their role goes beyond simply carrying out tasks: they play an active part in coordinating care, transmitting information and promoting inter-professional collaboration.

The pivotal role of the caregiver

The caregiver is in constant contact with the patient, enabling him/her to observe subtle changes in his/her state of health, needs and reactions to treatment. These observations are crucial, and must be communicated in a precise and timely fashion to the care team. For example, the detection of an increase in pain, the appearance of a new clinical sign or a change in the patient's mood can influence therapeutic decisions.

As a member of a multidisciplinary team, the nursing auxiliary collaborates with nurses, doctors, physiotherapists, dieticians, psychologists and social workers. This collaboration is based on fluid, respectful and professional communication, favoring comprehensive and coherent patient care.

The principles of effective communication

1. **Clarity and precision**: Information must be clear, concise and unambiguous. It is important to report the facts objectively, avoiding unfounded personal interpretations. For example, rather than saying "the patient is not well", it is preferable to specify "the patient has a temperature of 38.5°C, a heart rate of 100 bpm and complains of abdominal pain".

2. **Relevance**: It is essential to convey information that is relevant to the patient's care. This involves discerning what is important from what is less so, so as not to overwhelm the team with superfluous details.

3. **Timing**: Communication must be timely. Urgent or critical information should be transmitted immediately, while routine observations can be shared during transmissions or team meetings.

4. **Respect and courtesy**: Respectful communication fosters a climate of trust and collaboration. It's important to consider other professionals' points of view, listen attentively and express yourself courteously.

Communication tools

- **Oral transmissions**: These are key moments at the beginning and end of the shift, when essential patient information is shared. Nurses must take an active part, preparing in advance the important points to be discussed.

- **The patient record**: An essential tool for tracing care, it must be filled in rigorously. Notes must be legible, dated and signed, and must respect confidentiality.

- **Multidisciplinary meetings**: These provide an opportunity to discuss complex cases, draw up personalized care plans and share knowledge. The caregiver contributes by sharing observations and making suggestions.

- **Digital media**: The use of information technologies, such as care management software, facilitates real-time communication and data sharing. Caregivers need to be comfortable using these tools to access and update relevant information.

Interpersonal communication

- **Active listening**: This involves paying full attention to the speaker, showing interest in what he or she is saying, asking questions to clarify and rephrasing to check understanding.

- **Empathy**: Understanding colleagues' emotions and perspectives fosters deeper communication and better collaboration. This strengthens team bonds and creates a harmonious working environment.

- **Assertiveness**: Expressing yourself honestly and directly, while respecting others, is crucial to avoiding misunderstandings and frustrations. Caregivers need to feel comfortable sharing their opinions, asking questions or expressing concerns.

Managing communication barriers

There are several obstacles to effective communication:

- **Differences in terminology**: Professionals sometimes use technical terms specific to their discipline. It's important to clarify unfamiliar terms and use accessible language whenever possible.

- **Interpersonal conflicts**: Tensions may arise within the team. It is essential to deal with them constructively, giving priority to dialogue and the search for common solutions.

- **Workload**: Stress and fatigue can affect the quality of communication. Taking regular breaks and managing time effectively helps maintain an optimal level of communication.

The importance of non-verbal communication

Communication isn't just about words. Facial expressions, body language, tone of voice and eye contact play a major role in conveying messages. Caregivers need to be aware of their own non-verbal communication, and attentive to that of others, as it can reveal feelings not expressed verbally.

Working with families and friends

The patient's family and friends are often an integral part of the patient's care environment. Caregivers must communicate with them in a respectful manner, respecting professional secrecy and keeping them informed within the limits of their competence. Good communication with families contributes to their trust in the care team and to the patient's well-being.

Communication in emergency situations

In a medical emergency, communication must be fast, clear and effective. The orderly must :

- **Report the situation immediately**: Use emergency codes if necessary, inform colleagues first.

- **Provide precise information**: patient's identity, signs observed, actions already taken.

- **Coordinate actions**: work with the team to ensure an appropriate response, following established protocols.

Continuing education in communications

Developing communication skills is an ongoing process. Caregivers can take part in specific training courses, simulation workshops or debriefing sessions to improve their practice. Feedback and self-assessment are also valuable tools for progress.

The benefits of effective communication

- **For the patient**: better care coordination, personalized care, reduced risk of errors and improved satisfaction.

- **For the team**: stronger cohesion, increased efficiency, reduced stress and conflict.

- **For the caregiver**: A sense of self-esteem, a feeling of professional accomplishment and an opportunity for personal development.

- Management of medical tools and equipment

In the Internal Medicine department, the management of medical tools and equipment is an essential component of the nursing auxiliary's work. Proper use, rigorous maintenance and in-depth knowledge of medical devices contribute not only to the quality of care provided, but also to the safety of patients and nursing staff. This chapter explores the various aspects of medical equipment management, highlighting the caregiver's responsibilities in this field.

The importance of controlling medical equipment

Medical equipment is an indispensable tool for diagnosing, treating and monitoring patients. It encompasses a wide range of devices, from vital sign monitors and mobility equipment to infusion systems and respiratory assistance devices. Mastery of this equipment enables the nursing auxiliary to :

- **Ensuring efficient, precise care**: Correct use ensures that patients receive the right care at the right time.
- **Prevent errors linked to misuse**: knowledge of the equipment reduces the risk of potentially dangerous errors.
- **Ensuring patient safety**: Proper equipment management minimizes the risk of incidents or accidents.
- **Optimizing resources**: Efficient use of equipment contributes to cost management and equipment durability.

Equipment knowledge and training

A thorough knowledge of the equipment used in the department is essential. The orderly must be trained in :

- **How each device works**: Understand the basic principles, operating modes, possible settings and indications for which the equipment is used.

- **Operating procedures**: Know how to switch on, adjust, clean and switch off equipment in accordance with established protocols.

- **Safety measures**: Learn about the precautions to be taken to avoid electrical, mechanical or infectious risks associated with the use of equipment.

- **Recognizing malfunctions** : Be able to identify the signs of device failure or anomaly, and know what action to take in the event of a problem.

Training can be provided by experienced staff, biomedical engineers, or through training sessions organized by the facility. It's important to keep up to date with new technologies and updates to existing equipment.

Main equipment and management

1. **Vital signs monitors**
   Monitors enable continuous monitoring of vital parameters such as heart rate, blood pressure, oxygen saturation and respiratory rate.

   - **Correct use**: Check that sensors are correctly positioned, cables are in good condition and alarms are correctly set.
   - **Monitoring**: Pay attention to parameter variations and alarms, and know how to interpret the data displayed.
   - **Maintenance**: Clean sensors after each use, report any faults to technical service.

2. **Electric infusion pumps and syringes**
   These devices ensure precise administration of intravenous drugs and fluids.

   - **Programming**: Ensure that the dose, flow rate and volume to be infused are correctly programmed according to the medical prescription.
   - **Checks**: Regularly check that the pump is working properly, and monitor the injection site for signs of infiltration or phlebitis.

- ◦ **Safety**: Follow protocols to avoid infusion errors, such as overdosing or unexpected interruptions.

3. Oxygen therapy

Oxygen administration can be vital for patients suffering from respiratory failure.

- ◦ **Installation**: Know how to correctly install nasal cannula, oxygen masks or high-flow systems.
- ◦ **Settings**: Adjust flowmeter according to prescription, check oxygen levels in cylinders or centralized system regularly.
- ◦ **Monitoring**: Observe patient for signs of hypoxia or hyperoxia, monitor hydration of nasal mucosa.

4. Mobility and lifting devices

Medical beds, wheelchairs, lifts and other equipment facilitate patient mobilization.

- ◦ **Safe use**: Know how to move patients safely, avoiding falls or injuries.
- ◦ **Maintenance**: Check the condition of equipment before use, report any anomalies (e.g. defective brakes, worn straps).
- ◦ **Ergonomics**: Adjusting equipment for patient comfort and prevention of musculoskeletal disorders among caregivers.

5. Care and hygiene equipment

- ◦ **Sterilization and disinfection**: Ensure proper cleaning of reusable instruments, comply with sterilization protocols.
- ◦ **Inventory management**: Monitor consumable levels (gloves, gowns, single-use equipment), anticipate needs to avoid stock-outs.
- ◦ **Infection prevention** : Use single-use equipment in accordance with recommendations, dispose of medical waste through the appropriate channels.

Maintenance and incident reporting procedures

The nursing auxiliary must actively participate in the preventive maintenance of equipment:

- **Regular checks**: Check the condition of equipment before each use, and carry out functional tests if necessary.
- **Routine maintenance**: Clean equipment according to protocols, replace consumables (batteries, filters).
- **Reporting malfunctions**: In the event of a malfunction, label the device as out of order, remove it from the care circuit and inform the biomedical department.
- **Traceability**: Record work carried out on equipment in dedicated registers or software, to ensure tracking and regulatory compliance.

Safety and risk prevention

Managing medical equipment involves risks that need to be kept under control:

- **Electrical hazard**: check cable integrity, avoid overloading sockets, do not use damaged equipment.
- **Risk of infection**: Observe asepsis protocols, particularly for invasive equipment or equipment in contact with mucous membranes.
- **Risk of misuse**: Follow operating instructions carefully, do not improvise in case of doubt, seek advice from an experienced colleague.
- **Safety training**: Participate in training courses on equipment risk management and incident procedures (cardiac arrest, fire).

Optimizing equipment use

- **Rationalization**: Use equipment appropriately to avoid wasting resources, for example by putting appliances on standby when not in use.

- **Innovation**: Keep abreast of new technologies, participate in evaluations of new equipment, share feedback with the team.
- **Resource sharing**: coordinate with colleagues to use shared equipment, plan interventions to avoid conflicts of use.

Collaboration with the biomedical department

The biomedical department is a key partner in equipment management:

- **Communication**: Report problems promptly, provide precise information on the symptoms of the fault.
- **Feedback**: After maintenance work, test the device and confirm that it is working properly.
- **Participation in quality controls**: Assist technicians during periodic checks, facilitate access to equipment.

Raising awareness of regulatory aspects

Medical equipment is subject to strict standards:

- **Compliance**: Ensure that the equipment used complies with current standards and has been validated by the plant.
- **Documentation**: Knowledge of institutional protocols, user manuals and technical data sheets.
- **Data confidentiality and security**: For equipment storing patient data, ensure that information is protected, and comply with the establishment's IT security policies.

Involvement in continuous improvement

- **Feedback**: share difficulties encountered with the team, suggest improvements in equipment use or management.
- **Committee participation**: Participate in equipment working groups, contribute to the development of policies and procedures.

- **Training new arrivals**: Passing on knowledge and best practices to new staff members, ensuring quality supervision.

Chapter 3

Daily care in Internal Medicine

- Monitoring vital signs and clinical parameters

Monitoring vital signs and clinical parameters is an essential part of the role of the nursing auxiliary in internal medicine. It is a fundamental pillar of patient health assessment, enabling the early detection of signs of deterioration or improvement, and the adjustment of care accordingly. This rigorous monitoring contributes not only to patient safety, but also to the overall effectiveness of medical care.

The importance of monitoring vital signs

Vital signs are key indicators of the functioning of the body's physiological systems. They include body temperature, heart rate, blood pressure, respiratory rate and oxygen saturation. Regular monitoring of these parameters makes it possible to :

- **Detect abnormalities**: Quickly identify signs of infection, hemorrhage, cardiac or respiratory decompensation, among others.
- **Evaluate treatment effectiveness**: Check whether medical interventions, such as drug administration or oxygen therapy, are producing the expected effects.
- **Prevent complications**: Anticipate risks and implement appropriate preventive measures.
- **Inform the healthcare team**: Provide objective data to guide clinical decisions and adjust the care plan.

Techniques for measuring vital signs

1. Body temperature

- **Measurement methods**: Temperature can be measured buccally, axillary, rectally or tympanically. The choice of method depends on the patient's condition, age and institutional protocols.

- ◦ **Precautions**: Use a clean, calibrated thermometer, observe hygiene rules to avoid cross-infection, and ensure patient comfort.
- ◦ **Interpretation**: A temperature above 38°C indicates a fever, while a temperature below 36°C may indicate hypothermia. These variations require special attention.

2. Heart rate (pulse)

- ◦ **Methods**: Pulse can be measured at radial, carotid, femoral or apical level. Caregivers generally use the radial pulse for ease of access.
- ◦ **Technique**: Place two fingers (index and middle) on the artery, count the number of pulses for 60 seconds, note the rhythm (regular or irregular) and amplitude.
- ◦ **Interpretation**: Tachycardia (pulse > 100 bpm) or bradycardia (pulse < 60 bpm) may indicate an underlying pathology or drug effect.

3. Blood pressure

- ◦ **Measurement methods**: It can be measured manually with an aneroid tensiometer and stethoscope, or automatically with an electronic monitor.
- ◦ **Manual technique**: Place the cuff correctly on the arm, inflate the cuff to 20-30 mmHg above the expected pressure, deflate slowly and listen for Korotkoff sounds to determine systolic and diastolic pressures.
- ◦ **Precautions**: Make sure the patient is at rest, avoid measuring on an arm with a perfusion or arteriovenous fistula, use an appropriately sized cuff.

- ○ **Interpretation**: Hypertension or hypotension requires thorough evaluation and appropriate medical intervention.

4. Respiratory frequency

- ○ **Technique**: Observe thoracic or abdominal movements discreetly for one minute, to prevent the patient from voluntarily modifying his breathing.
- ○ **Interpretation**: Tachypnea (FR > 20/min) may indicate respiratory distress, infection or pain. Bradypnea (FR < 12/min) may be associated with central nervous system depression or the effect of certain drugs.

5. Oxygen saturation (SpO2)

- ○ **Using the pulse oximeter**: Place the sensor on a finger, earlobe or toe, making sure the area is clean and well perfused.
- ○ **Interpretation**: Saturations below 95% may indicate hypoxemia. Measurements below 90% require immediate intervention.
- ○ **Precautions**: Check that the sensor is correctly positioned, avoid interference (dark nail polish, excessive movement), ensure that the device is calibrated.

Monitoring of other clinical parameters

1. Capillary blood glucose

- ○ **Indications** : Particularly important in patients with diabetes or at risk of hypoglycemia/ hyperglycemia.
- ○ **Technique**: After disinfecting the puncture site (usually the fingertip), prick with a sterile lancet

and collect a drop of blood on the test strip inserted in the glucometer.

- ○ **Precautions** : Use single-use equipment, observe hygiene rules, handle waste according to protocols.
- ○ **Interpretation**: Normal fasting blood glucose levels are between 0.70 and 1.10 g/L. Values outside these limits require intervention.

2. Diuresis

- ○ **Significance**: Measuring the amount of urine excreted enables assessment of renal function, fluid balance and response to certain treatments (diuretics).
- ○ **Technique**: Collect urine over a set period, usually 24 hours, using graduated containers.
- ○ **Precautions**: Inform patient of procedure, ensure privacy, handle samples with gloves.
- ○ **Interpretation**: Oliguria (diuresis < 500 mL/24h) or anuria (diuresis < 100 mL/24h) is cause for concern and should be reported.

3. Pain assessment

- ○ **Use of scales**: Numerical scale (0 to 10), simple verbal scale, visual analog scale or scales adapted to non-communicative patients.
- ○ **Importance**: Pain is a subjective but essential parameter, influencing the patient's quality of life and recovery.
- ○ **Intervention**: Note intensity, location, nature (acute, chronic), aggravating or relieving factors, and inform team for appropriate management.

4. Observation of general condition

- ○ **Awareness and orientation**: Assess whether the patient is alert, oriented in time and space, and able to respond to stimuli.
- ○ **Skin and mucous membrane discoloration**: look for signs of cyanosis, pallor, jaundice or rash.
- ○ **Hydration and nutrition**: Note signs of dehydration (dry mucous membranes, skin folds) or undernutrition (weight loss, muscle wasting).
- ○ **Digestive and intestinal function**: Monitor nausea, vomiting, appetite, intestinal transit, stool appearance.

Documentation and communication of observations

- **Traceability**: accurately record measured values in the patient file, indicating date, time and any relevant observations.
- **Reporting abnormalities**: Inform the nurse or doctor immediately of any abnormal parameters or significant changes.
- **Continuity of care**: Pass on information at shift changeovers, highlighting points of attention for follow-up.

Precautions and best practices

- **Standardization of techniques**: Follow established protocols to ensure measurement reliability and data comparability.
- **Hygiene and asepsis**: Use clean or sterile devices, disinfect equipment as recommended, wash hands before and after each patient.
- **Respect for the patient**: Explain procedures, obtain consent, ensure comfort and privacy, adapt techniques to the patient's abilities.

- **Continuing education**: Keep abreast of technological developments and new recommendations in clinical monitoring.

The caregiver's proactive role

- **Anticipation**: Be aware of the patient's risk factors (history, current treatments) to target monitoring.
- **Global observation**: Don't just look at the numbers, interpret the signs by placing them in their clinical context.
- **Collaboration**: Work in close coordination with the care team, share information and participate in clinical discussions.
- **Patient education**: inform patients of the importance of monitoring, involve them in follow-up, encourage them to report their symptoms.

Special cases

- **Critical patients**: In unstable patients, the frequency of measurements must be increased, and the caregiver must be ready to react quickly.
- **Non-communicative patients**: Adapt assessment techniques, use indirect methods and be alert to non-verbal signs.
- **Pediatric and geriatric patients**: take age-related specificities into account, adjust monitoring methods and intervals.

- Assistance with nursing procedures

The nursing auxiliary plays a fundamental role in the Internal Medicine care team, not only in the day-to-day care of patients, but also in providing invaluable assistance with nursing procedures. This close collaboration between the orderly and the nurse is essential to guarantee quality care, ensure continuity of care and meet the complex needs of hospitalized patients. This chapter explores in depth the caregiver's role in assisting with nursing procedures, highlighting the skills required, the responsibilities shared and the impact on the patient's care pathway.

Complementary roles for caregivers and nurses

In internal medicine, patients often present with multiple pathologies requiring specific interventions and constant monitoring. The nurse is responsible for care planning, treatment administration, clinical assessment and coordination with other healthcare professionals. The nursing auxiliary supports the nurse by carrying out essential tasks, enabling him or her to lighten the workload and concentrate on more technical procedures.

This complementarity is based on a mutual understanding of roles, effective communication and respect for each other's skills. The nursing auxiliary must know the limits of its field of intervention, act under the delegation of the nurse and respect established protocols.

Areas of nursing assistance

1. **Preparing equipment and the environment**
   The nursing auxiliary plays a key role in preparing the materials needed for nursing procedures. This includes :

   - **Equipment assembly**: Prepare treatment trays, sterilize instruments if necessary, check availability of consumables (compresses, syringes, gloves, etc.).
   - **Space planning**: Organize the environment to facilitate the procedure, ensure the cleanliness and asepsis of the care area, adjust the patient's bed to the appropriate height.

○ **Anticipating needs**: Plan specific equipment according to the procedures planned (e.g. ECG, perfusion, puncture).

2. Technical care support

During nursing procedures, the nursing auxiliary provides direct assistance in a number of ways:

○ **Patient positioning**: Help the patient adopt the right position for care, ensure comfort and safety, use appropriate mobilization techniques.

○ **Maintaining asepsis**: Ensure compliance with hygiene rules, for example by limiting sources of contamination and handling equipment with care.

○ **Psychological support**: Reassuring the patient, explaining the course of treatment if necessary, being there to soothe anxieties or discomfort.

○ **Observation**: Monitor the patient's reactions during the procedure, and report any abnormalities (intense pain, discomfort, bleeding) immediately.

3. After-care and follow-up

After the nursing act, the nursing auxiliary contributes to the patient's follow-up:

○ **Cleaning and storage**: Dispose of waste according to protocols, disinfect reusable materials, store equipment.

○ **Post-procedure monitoring**: Observe vital signs, check puncture or injection site for complications (hematoma, infection), report observations to the nurse.

○ **Patient comfort**: Resettle the patient in a comfortable position, make sure they have access to their personal belongings, offer water or a snack if authorized.

Practical examples of nursing assistance

1. Intravenous drug administration

- ◦ **Preparation**: The caregiver prepares the necessary equipment (infusion set, solution, infusion pump), checks expiration dates and labels solutions if necessary.
- ◦ **Assistance during insertion**: Helps the nurse by holding the patient's limb, ensuring good visibility of the vein site.
- ◦ **Monitoring**: After insertion, monitor the infusion flow rate, observe the site for signs of infiltration or phlebitis, inform the nurse of any abnormalities.

2. Blood sampling

- ◦ **Preparing the patient**: Informs the patient of the treatment to come, makes sure he/she is in a comfortable position, exposes the puncture site.
- ◦ **Support during sampling**: Holds equipment at nurse's disposal, applies tourniquet if requested, supports patient in case of apprehension.
- ◦ **Post-test follow-up**: Apply compression to the site, place a dressing, monitor for hematoma.

3. Complex wound care

- ◦ **Preparing the sterile field**: Place sterile instruments and dressings on the tray, observing asepsis rules.
- ◦ **Active assistance**: Can help cut dressings, hold non-sterile instruments, reposition the patient during care.
- ◦ **Patient education**: reinforces the nurse's explanations of home care and signs to look out for.

Skills required to assist with nursing procedures

- **Knowledge of protocols**: The nursing auxiliary must master procedures relating to nursing acts to ensure effective and safe assistance.
- **Dexterity and precision**: Handling medical equipment requires manual dexterity and attention to detail.
- **Clear communication**: Optimum coordination with the nurse requires fluid communication, the ability to understand instructions quickly and to report relevant information.
- **Empathy and patience**: Understand the patient's needs and be gentle, especially during potentially painful or anxiety-provoking procedures.
- **Reactivity**: Being able to react promptly to unexpected events, complications or changes in the patient's condition.

The limits of the caregiver's role

It is crucial to respect the legal and ethical limits of the profession. Caregivers may not carry out acts reserved for nurses, such as administering injectable drugs, inserting venous catheters or performing specific dressings without appropriate delegation. All assistance must be provided under the nurse's supervision, in compliance with the establishment's protocols and guidelines.

The importance of ongoing training

Medical practices are constantly evolving, and caregivers need to keep their knowledge up to date to remain effective in their caring role. Participating in training courses, practical workshops and information sessions enables them to :

- **Improving technical skills**: discovering new methods, familiarizing yourself with innovative equipment.
- **Keeping abreast of new regulations**: Keeping abreast of legal developments concerning healthcare procedures.

- **Strengthen collaboration**: share experiences with colleagues, harmonize practices within the team.

Benefits for the patient

The caregiver's assistance with nursing acts has a direct impact on the quality of care:

- **Smoother care**: procedures are carried out more efficiently, reducing waiting times for patients.
- **Increased safety**: the double vigilance of the nurse and caregiver minimizes the risk of errors or complications.
- **A relationship of trust**: the caregiver's reassuring presence promotes the patient's well-being, and reduces the anxiety associated with medical procedures.

Enhancing the role of the caregiver

Recognizing the importance of the caregiver in assisting with nursing procedures is essential for :

- **Reinforce motivation**: Recognition of work accomplished encourages commitment and job satisfaction.
- **Promote teamwork**: harmonious collaboration improves the working atmosphere and efficiency of the department.
- **Developing skills**: Offering opportunities for training and responsibility contributes to professional fulfillment.

- Pain management and patient comfort

Pain management and patient comfort are essential components of care in Internal Medicine. Patients admitted to this department often present with complex pathologies, associated with painful symptoms and physical or psychological discomfort. The caregiver plays a key role in assessing and relieving pain, and in improving the patient's overall well-being. This chapter explores approaches and techniques to ensure optimal pain and comfort management, while respecting medical protocols and individual patient needs.

Understanding pain

Pain is a subjective sensory and emotional experience associated with actual or potential tissue damage. It can be acute or chronic, nociceptive or neuropathic, and is influenced by physiological, psychological and socio-cultural factors. In internal medicine, patients may suffer from pain related to their illness, medical interventions or co-morbidities. It is crucial for the caregiver to understand the mechanisms of pain in order to better assess and respond appropriately.

Pain assessment

Accurate pain assessment is the first step towards effective pain management. Caregivers must use validated tools to measure the intensity, quality, location and evolution of pain.

- **Assessment scales**: Use scales adapted to the patient, such as the numerical scale (0 to 10), the visual analog scale, or the simple verbal scale. For non-communicative patients, the behavioral scale (Doloplus, Algoplus) can be used.

- **Pain history**: Ask the patient about the characteristics of his or her pain (onset, duration, aggravating or relieving factors, impact on daily activities).

- **Observation**: Pay attention to non-verbal signs of pain, such as grimaces, agitation, tachycardia, high blood pressure, or behavioral changes.

The caregiver's role in pain management

The caregiver intervenes on several levels to relieve the patient's pain:

1. Administration of analgesic treatments

- ○ **Prescription compliance**: Although medication administration is generally reserved for the nurse, the orderly can help prepare the patient, check his or her identity, and ensure compliance.

- ○ **Monitoring effects**: Observe the effects of analgesic treatments, report any ineffectiveness or appearance of undesirable effects (drowsiness, nausea, constipation, respiratory depression).

2. Non-pharmacological pain relief techniques

- ○ **Application of heat or cold**: Use hot compresses to relax muscles or ice packs to reduce inflammation, respecting contraindications and precautions for use.

- ○ **Massages and gentle mobilizations**: Perform light massages to improve blood circulation and muscle relaxation, avoiding painful or sensitive areas.

- ○ **Relaxation and distraction**: Encourage relaxation techniques such as deep breathing and guided meditation, or offer distracting activities (music, reading, conversation).

3. Positioning and environment

- ○ **Comfortable positioning**: Help the patient adopt an analgesic position, using pillows, cushions or specific supports to relieve pressure points.

- ○ **Adapting the environment**: Ensure that the room is quiet, with a pleasant temperature and adequate lighting, and that the patient has access to personal comforting items.

4. Patient education and information

- ○ **Explaining care**: Informing patients about upcoming procedures and prescribed treatments, to reduce anxiety and pain perception.

- ○ **Encouraging expression**: Invite patients to verbalize their pain, fears and expectations, so that care can be adapted to their specific needs.

Managing overall patient comfort

Beyond physical pain, patient comfort encompasses psychological, emotional and social well-being.

- **Personalized hygiene care**: Provide hygiene care that respects the patient's preferences and is attentive to his or her modesty and dignity.

- **Adapted nutrition**: Ensure that food is provided in accordance with prescribed diets, while taking into account the patient's tastes, chewing and swallowing abilities.

- **Promoting sleep**: Encourage rest by limiting nocturnal interruptions, reducing noise and creating an atmosphere conducive to sleep.

- **Psychological support**: listening, empathizing, offering a reassuring presence, especially for isolated or anxious patients.

Collaboration with the multidisciplinary team

Managing pain and patient comfort is a shared responsibility within the healthcare team.

- **Effective communication**: Pass on observations on pain and patient comfort during communications, immediately report urgent situations or significant changes.

- **Participation in meetings**: Contribute to discussions on the care plan, propose ideas to improve patient well-being, share feedback.

- **Coordinating interventions**: working in synergy with nurses, physiotherapists, psychologists and dieticians, to provide comprehensive, coherent care.

Personalized approach to pain

Every patient is unique, and the perception of pain is influenced by cultural, spiritual and personal factors.

- **Respect for beliefs**: Take into account the patient's religious or cultural convictions when managing pain, for example by respecting their preferences in terms of treatments or complementary practices.

- **Adapting to cognitive abilities**: For patients with cognitive impairments or communication difficulties, adapt pain assessment and relief methods.

- **Involving loved ones**: Working with family or caregivers to better understand the patient, boost morale and reinforce a sense of security.

Preventing pain-related complications

Poorly controlled pain can lead to physiological and psychological complications.

- **Preventing chronicity**: Act quickly to relieve acute pain and prevent it from becoming long-lasting.

- **Side-effect monitoring**: Be alert to complications associated with analgesic treatments, such as constipation, impaired alertness and the risk of falling.

- **Encouraging mobilization**: Encouraging adapted physical activity to prevent joint stiffness and muscle wasting, and improve patient morale.

Ongoing training and knowledge updating

Pain management is evolving with medical advances and new therapeutic approaches.

- **Skills updating**: Participate in training courses on pain management, non-pharmacological techniques and complementary approaches.

- **Professional watch**: Keep abreast of recommendations, institutional protocols and innovations in the field of pain management.

- **Sharing best practices**: exchanging successful experiences and challenges with colleagues to enrich professional practices.

Ethics and respect for patient choice

Pain management must respect patients' rights and wishes.

- **Informed consent**: Ensures that the patient understands pain relief options and respects his or her choice to accept or refuse certain treatments.

- **Confidentiality**: Protect the patient's personal information, particularly concerning pain and comfort.

- **Autonomy**: Encouraging patients to take an active part in their own care, valuing their abilities and supporting their independence.

Special cases: pain at the end of life

In internal medicine, some patients are in a palliative or end-of-life phase. Pain and comfort management take on a special dimension.

- **Maximum relief**: Prioritize pain control, even if this means high doses of analgesics, in compliance with protocols and advance directives.

- **All-round support**: offering emotional and spiritual support, being there for the patient and family, facilitating goodbyes and moments of intimacy.

- **Respecting patients' wishes**: Taking into account patients' wishes regarding their end-of-life care, working with the team to ensure that care is provided in accordance with their values.

- Prevention of pressure sores and nosocomial infections
The prevention of pressure sores and nosocomial infections is a crucial component of the role of the nursing auxiliary in internal medicine. These two issues represent major challenges for the quality of care and safety of hospitalized patients. Pressure sores, also known as pressure ulcers, are skin lesions caused by prolonged immobilization, while nosocomial infections are hospital-acquired infections that are often resistant to antibiotics. The caregiver, through his or her proximity to the patient and knowledge of care protocols, plays a key role in preventing these complications. This chapter explores strategies and best practices for effectively preventing pressure sores and nosocomial infections, thereby helping to improve patient prognosis and comfort.

Understanding pressure sores: mechanisms and risk factors

Pressure sores form as a result of prolonged pressure on an area of the body, leading to tissue ischemia and necrosis. They occur mainly in patients who are bedridden, immobile or have sensitivity problems. The areas most affected are bony points of support, such as the sacrum, heels, trochanters and malleoli.

Several factors increase the risk of developing pressure sores:

- **Immobility**: Patients in bed, wheelchairs or with reduced mobility.
- **Nutritional disorders**: malnutrition, dehydration, protein deficiencies.
- **Altered consciousness**: Coma, sedation, neurological disorders.
- **Incontinence**: Skin moisture promotes maceration.
- **Advanced age**: fragile skin, loss of elasticity, associated comorbidities.

The caregiver's role in pressure sore prevention

1. **Risk assessment**
   The nursing auxiliary participates in the initial and ongoing assessment of pressure sore risk, using specific scales such as the Norton or Braden scales. This assessment enables high-risk patients to be identified and appropriate preventive measures to be put in place.

2. **Regular mobilization**

   - **Position changes**: Alternate patient positions every two hours, respecting rotation patterns to relieve pressure points.
   - **Use of technical aids**: Anti-decubitus mattresses, positioning cushions, heel supports, which distribute pressure and reduce the risk of injury.

- ○ **Encourage active mobilization**: Encourage patients to move around, perform simple exercises and participate in transfers if possible.

3. Skin care

- ○ **Rigorous hygiene**: cleanse skin with mild products, dry carefully without rubbing, especially in skin folds.
- ○ **Skin hydration**: Apply moisturizing creams to maintain skin elasticity, avoiding irritating or allergenic products.
- ○ **Monitoring at-risk areas**: Inspect contact areas daily, looking for redness, indurations, signs of maceration or incipient lesions.

4. Incontinence management

- ○ **Skin protection**: Use skin barriers or protective creams to prevent irritation from urine or feces.
- ○ **Frequent changes**: Replace soiled incontinence pads promptly, and ensure intimate hygiene after each incontinence episode.
- ○ **Moisture prevention**: Keep skin dry, avoid moisture-retaining synthetic undergarments.

5. Nutrition and hydration

- ○ **Intake monitoring**: Ensure that the patient's diet is rich in proteins, vitamins and minerals essential for healing.
- ○ **Adequate hydration**: Encourage regular fluid intake, watch for signs of dehydration.
- ○ **Collaboration with the dietician**: Adapting diets to the patient's specific needs.

6. Patient and family education

- ◦ **Awareness**: Explain the risks of pressure sores, the importance of mobilization and skin care.
- ◦ **Involvement**: Involve the patient in preventive measures, show him how to change position, massage at-risk areas.
- ◦ **Support for family and friends**: Train the family in preventive actions, especially with a view to returning home.

Understanding nosocomial infections: issues and transmission

Nosocomial infections are hospital-acquired infections, often caused by antibiotic-resistant bacteria. They can affect various sites: urinary tract, surgical site, lungs (pneumonia), bloodstream (septicemia). Modes of transmission include :

- **Direct contact**: Between nursing staff and patient, via contaminated hands.
- **Indirect contact**: via medical equipment, contaminated surfaces.
- **Airborne transmission**: For certain pathogens, via droplets or aerosols.

Vulnerable patients are those with weakened immune defenses, carriers of invasive devices (catheters, probes), or undergoing aggressive treatments.

The caregiver's role in preventing nosocomial infections

1. Hand hygiene

- ◦ **Appropriate technique**: Use hydro-alcoholic friction or soap washing as indicated, respecting the WHO's five key moments:
  - ▪ Before touching a patient.
  - ▪ Before an aseptic procedure.
  - ▪ After exposure to biological fluids.
  - ▪ After touching a patient.

69

- After touching the patient's environment.
  - **Sufficient time**: Ensure rubbing or washing for at least 30 seconds for optimum effectiveness.
  - **Hygiene promotion**: Make colleagues and patients aware of the importance of this measure.

2. Use of personal protective equipment (PPE)

  - **Gloves**: Wear non-sterile gloves for treatments involving exposure to biological fluids, and change them between patients.
  - **Gowns, masks, goggles**: Use according to additional precautions (contact, droplets, air) depending on the infectious risk.
  - **Safe removal**: Remove PPE without contaminating clothing or skin, dispose of waste through appropriate channels.

3. Environmental maintenance

  - **Surface cleaning**: Regularly disinfect surfaces that come into frequent contact (tables, bed rails, handles).
  - **Equipment management**: Clean and disinfect reusable equipment, use single-use equipment whenever possible.
  - **Linen and waste**: Handle soiled linen with care, place in special bags, manage infectious waste in accordance with protocols.

4. Precautions during invasive care

  - **Asepsis**: Observe asepsis rules when caring for catheters, urinary catheters and drains.
  - **Minimal handling**: limit handling of invasive devices, avoid unnecessary disconnections.

- ○ **Site monitoring**: Observe insertion points for signs of infection (redness, warmth, pain, discharge).

5. Vaccinations and employee health

- ○ **Up-to-date vaccinations**: Make sure your vaccinations are up to date (hepatitis B, flu) to protect yourself and your patients.
- ○ **State of health**: Do not report to work if you have a contagious disease, report accidental exposure to infectious agents.

6. Training and awareness-raising

- ○ **Updating knowledge**: Participate in training courses on hospital hygiene and new recommendations.
- ○ **Information sharing**: Communicate with the team on risk situations, incidents and corrective measures.
- ○ **Safety culture**: Encourage a proactive attitude to infection prevention, report shortcomings, suggest improvements.

Synergy between pressure sore and nosocomial infection prevention

Measures to prevent pressure sores and nosocomial infections are often interconnected. For example:

- **Skin care**: Maintaining skin integrity reduces the risk of infection, as damaged skin is a gateway for pathogens.
- **Hygiene during care**: Apply the principles of asepsis when dressing pressure sores to avoid superinfection.
- **Safe mobilization**: Use appropriate lifting techniques to avoid injury, limit unnecessary contact with the patient carrying a transmissible infection.

Involving patients in prevention

It is important to involve patients in their own safety:

- **Information**: Explain the measures taken to prevent pressure sores and infections, the reasons for them and the benefits.
- **Active participation**: Encourage patients to report any discomfort, pain, redness or signs of infection.
- **Personal hygiene**: If possible, help patients to maintain adequate personal hygiene, and provide them with the means to wash their hands.

Managing special situations

- **Immunocompromised patients**: Reinforce protective measures, limit visits, use extra precautions.
- **Nosocomial epidemics**: In the event of an epidemic (e.g. influenza, gastroenteritis), apply specific guidelines, participate in screening, isolate infected patients.

Chapter 4

Helping the patient

- Establishing therapeutic communication

Therapeutic communication is a fundamental element of patient care in internal medicine. It is much more than a simple exchange of information; it is an essential tool for establishing a relationship of trust, understanding the patient's deepest needs and supporting them throughout their care. For the caregiver, developing effective therapeutic communication is both an art and a professional skill, requiring empathy, active listening, respect and understanding of interpersonal dynamics.

The importance of therapeutic communication

Therapeutic communication aims to promote patient well-being, encourage engagement in care and improve clinical outcomes. It enables :

- **Creating a relationship of trust**: By establishing a sincere bond with the patient, the caregiver reduces anxiety, increases cooperation and facilitates the sharing of important information.
- **Understanding the patient's needs**: Beyond physical symptoms, patients may have emotional, social or spiritual concerns that influence their health.
- **Facilitating adherence to treatment**: Good communication helps to explain procedures, answer questions and reassure patients, thereby improving adherence to prescribed treatments.
- **Detecting non-verbal cues**: Facial expressions, tone of voice and body language can reveal vital information about the patient's condition.

The fundamental principles of therapeutic communication

1. **Active listening**
   Active listening is a key skill that involves paying full

attention to the patient, understanding their message, interpreting their emotions and responding appropriately. This includes:

- **Focus on the patient**: Avoid distractions, maintain eye contact, adopt an open posture.
- **Encourage expression**: Use verbal prompts like "I'm listening", "Can you tell me more?", and head nods.
- **Reformulate**: Repeat or paraphrase what the patient has said to check understanding.
- **Clarify**: Ask open-ended questions to deepen understanding, e.g. "How do you feel about this?".

2. Empathy

Empathy means putting yourself in the patient's shoes, understanding their feelings and perspectives without judgment. It manifests itself through :

- **Acknowledging the patient's emotions**: "I can see that this worries you a lot."
- **Express compassion**: "I'm sorry you're going through this."
- **Avoid judgment**: Welcome the patient's feelings without criticism or prejudice.

3. Respect and dignity

Every patient deserves to be treated with respect, whatever their condition. This means :

- **Use the patient's preferred name**: Ask what they would like to be called.
- **Respect confidentiality**: Ensure that shared information remains private.
- **Taking preferences into account**: Respecting patients' choices regarding their care, wherever possible.

4. **Congruence and authenticity** Being authentic in communication means being sincere and transparent. Caregivers must be consistent between what they say and what they express non-verbally.

   ○ **Avoid pretense**: Don't pretend to understand if you don't.
   ○ **Be honest**: Provide accurate information, even if it's hard to hear, while respecting your professional role.
   ○ **Demonstrate integrity**: Act in accordance with ethical and professional values.

5. **Adapting to the patient**
   Every patient is unique, with his or her own needs, beliefs and communication skills. The caregiver must adapt his or her approach according to :

   ○ **Age**: Adapting language and approach for children, adults or the elderly.
   ○ **Culture and language**: Take cultural differences into account, using interpreters if necessary.
   ○ **Cognitive skills**: Adapt communication for patients with cognitive disorders, using simple sentences and repeating if necessary.

Therapeutic communication techniques

1. **Open-ended questions**
   Open-ended questions encourage patients to express themselves freely and provide detailed information.

   ○ **Examples**: "How would you describe your pain?", "What's worrying you most right now?"
   ○ **Advantages**: They allow you to explore the patient's feelings, perceptions and experiences.

76

2. Therapeutic silence

Silence can be a powerful tool for enabling patients to reflect and express themselves at their own pace.

- ○ **How to use**: After a patient's question or emotional statement, leave a moment of silence to allow them to elaborate their thoughts.
- ○ **Caution**: The silence must be comfortable, without pressure, and the caregiver must remain present and attentive.

3. Validation

Validation involves recognizing and accepting the patient's feelings.

- ○ **Examples**: "It's understandable that you feel anxious in this situation."
- ○ **Effect**: Reinforces confidence and the feeling of being understood.

4. Focusing

Help patients focus on a particular subject, especially if they are scattered or confused.

- ○ **Technique**: "Let's talk a little more about what's worrying you about your treatment."
- ○ **Purpose**: To facilitate clarification of concerns and care planning.

5. Information

Providing patients with clear, appropriate information to help them understand their situation and care.

- ○ **Examples**: Explaining a procedure, the possible side effects of a drug.
- ○ **Importance**: Promotes patient autonomy and reduces anxiety linked to the unknown.

Barriers to therapeutic communication

There are several obstacles to effective communication:

- **Technical language**: Using complex medical terms can confuse the patient. Simple, clear language is preferable.
- **Judgment or prejudice** : Avoid letting your own opinions influence communication.
- **Environmental distractions**: Noise, frequent interruptions and lack of privacy can disrupt communication.
- **Patient's emotional state**: Pain, fear and anger can affect the patient's ability to communicate. It's important to recognize these emotions and deal with them sensitively.

Strategies for improving communication

- **Create a supportive environment**: find a quiet place, ensure confidentiality, sit at the patient's level.
- **Use non-verbal language**: smiles, nods, open posture to show interest and support.
- **Avoid interruptions**: Allow patients to finish sentences, don't rush them.
- **Adapt the pace**: Speak slowly, giving the patient time to understand and respond.
- **Check comprehension**: Ask the patient to rephrase what has been said to make sure he or she has understood.

The caregiver's role in interdisciplinary communication

Therapeutic communication is not limited to interaction with the patient, but also extends to collaboration with the care team.

- **Effective communication**: Communicate important information gathered from the patient to nurses and doctors.
- **Sharing observations**: Report changes in the patient's condition, concerns or specific needs.

- **Care coordination**: Participate in team meetings, contribute to individualized care plans.

Special cases: difficult or vulnerable patients

- **Aggressive or hostile patients**: Remain calm, don't take behavior personally, try to understand the causes of distress.
- **Non-communicative patients**: Use visual aids, gestures and facial expressions to communicate.
- **Patients at the end of life**: offering a silent presence, being receptive to emotional and spiritual needs, supporting loved ones.

Continuing education in therapeutic communication

Developing communication skills is an ongoing process.

- **Self-evaluation**: Reflect on your own practices, identify strengths and areas for improvement.
- **Training**: Participate in workshops and seminars on communication and patient psychology.
- **Supervision**: Ask experienced colleagues for feedback, share complex situations.

The impact of therapeutic communication on patient experience

By establishing effective therapeutic communication, the caregiver plays a key role in improving the patient experience. By reducing anxiety, promoting a better understanding of the disease and its treatment, and strengthening the patient's commitment to care, they contribute directly to better clinical outcomes. Quality communication can also reduce the risk of medical errors, improve patient compliance and increase overall patient satisfaction.

- Psychological support and guidance

Providing psychological support and guidance to patients is an essential part of the role of the nursing auxiliary in Internal Medicine. Patients hospitalized in this department are often faced with serious, chronic or complex illnesses, which can give rise to feelings of anxiety, fear, sadness or discouragement. The caregiver, with his or her constant presence and humane approach, is ideally placed to provide effective psychological support, promote the patient's mental well-being and contribute to his or her overall recovery.

Understanding the psychological impact of illness

The disease affects not only the body, but also the mind and emotions. Patients may experience :

- **Anxiety** about uncertain diagnosis, treatment or prognosis.
- **Depression** due to loss of autonomy, physical limitations or social isolation.
- **Anger or frustration** in reaction to the illness itself or to hospital constraints.
- **Fear** of pain, death or invasive medical procedures.
- **Feelings of powerlessness** in the face of dependence and medical control.

Understanding these emotions is essential to adapting support and accompaniment appropriately.

The caregiver's role in psychological support

1. **A caring presence**

   The caregiver's simple presence can bring comfort and security to the patient. By being available and attentive, he or she creates a bond of trust that facilitates the expression of feelings.

   ◦ **Active listening**: Paying full attention to the patient, without interruption or judgment, to understand his or her deepest concerns.

- **Empathy**: Showing understanding and sensitivity to the patient's emotions, demonstrating sincere compassion.
- **Respect**: Treat patients with dignity, respecting their values, beliefs and privacy.

2. Encouraging the expression of feelings

It's important to allow patients to freely express their emotions, fears and doubts.

- **Open-ended questions**: Ask questions that encourage dialogue, such as "How are you feeling today?" or "What's on your mind most right now?".
- **Emotional validation**: Recognize and accept the patient's feelings, avoiding minimizing or denying them.
- **Therapeutic silence**: Respect moments of silence, which may be necessary for the patient to reflect or gather his thoughts.

3. Providing clear, reassuring information

The unknown can be a major source of anxiety. The caregiver can help reduce this uncertainty.

- **Simple explanations**: Provide information on procedures, care or the course of the day, in understandable terms.
- **Clarifying doubts**: Answer patients' questions or refer them to the appropriate professional if necessary.
- **Preparing for procedures**: Inform patients in advance of upcoming treatments or examinations, to reduce surprise and apprehension.

4. Supporting autonomy and self-esteem

Encouraging patients to take an active part in their care can improve their morale and sense of control.

- Involvement in decision-making: Involve patients in choices concerning their day-to-day care, wherever possible.
- Positive reinforcement: Valorize patients' efforts and progress, however small, to boost their self-confidence.
- Adapted activities: Suggest activities that match the patient's interests and abilities, to keep them engaged and enjoying themselves.

5. Managing stress and anxiety

The caregiver can suggest simple techniques to help the patient manage stress.

- Relaxation techniques: Teach deep breathing, muscle relaxation or guided meditation exercises.
- Soothing environment: Create a calm, comfortable environment by reducing noise pollution and ensuring adequate lighting.
- Positive distraction: Offer magazines, books, music or games to divert the patient's attention from preoccupations.

6. Support for loved ones

Family and friends play a crucial role in the patient's psychological support.

- Open communication: Facilitating dialogue between patients and their families, while respecting confidentiality and the patient's wishes.
- Resource referral: Inform families about available support services, such as discussion groups or social services.
- Emotional support for loved ones: listening to the concerns of families, who may also experience anxiety or distress.

Specific techniques for effective support

- **Active listening**: Focusing fully on the patient, using verbal and non-verbal cues to show commitment.
- **Rephrasing**: Repeating or paraphrasing the patient's words to show understanding and clarify messages.
- **Avoid judgment**: Welcome the patient's feelings without criticism or moralizing.
- **Language adaptation**: Use simple terms, avoid medical jargon, make sure the patient understands the information.
- **Respecting the patient's rhythm**: Don't force the patient to talk or participate, and respect his or her moments of silence or withdrawal.

Psychological support in special situations

1. Patients at the end of life

- ○ **Compassionate care**: Being present, listening without reserve, respecting the patient's wishes regarding their dignity and comfort.
- ○ **Spiritual support**: Facilitate access to a chaplain or spiritual advisor if the patient so desires.
- ○ **Pain management**: Collaborate with the team to ensure optimal relief of physical symptoms.

2. Patients with cognitive disorders

- ○ **Adapted communication**: Use short sentences, repetition, visual aids if necessary.
- ○ **Safe environment**: Maintain temporal and spatial reference points, avoid sudden changes in routine.
- ○ **Appropriate stimulation**: Offer simple activities that encourage cognitive stimulation without causing frustration.

3. Adolescent and young adult patients

- ○ **Respect for individuality**: Recognize age-related needs, such as the desire for autonomy and privacy.
- ○ **Supporting social relationships**: Helping to maintain ties with friends and peers.
- ○ **Sensitivity to concerns**: Tactfully address topics such as body image, sexuality or professional future.

Coordination with the multidisciplinary team

- **Effective communication**: Share observations on the patient's psychological state with the team, while respecting confidentiality.
- **Participation in department meetings**: Contribute to discussions on the care plan, suggest appropriate interventions.
- **Referral to specialized professionals**: If necessary, suggest the intervention of a psychologist, psychiatrist or social worker.

Taking care of yourself as a caregiver

Psychological support can be emotionally demanding. It's important that caregivers take care of themselves too.

- **Stress management**: using relaxation techniques, maintaining work-life balance.
- **Supervision and support**: Discuss difficult situations with colleagues or superiors, take part in discussion groups.

- **Continuing education**: Training in communication techniques, emotional management and relevant therapeutic approaches.

Case study: Supporting a depressed patient

A patient has just learned that his chronic illness has worsened. He expresses sadness, says he feels useless and has lost hope.

- **Empathetic listening**: The caregiver sits close to the patient, listens without interrupting, shows understanding.
- **Validation of feelings**: "I understand that this news is difficult to accept."
- **Encouraging expression**: "Would you like to talk more about it?"
- **Support proposal**: "I'm here to help you. If you'd like, I can talk to the nurse so we can see together how we can support you."
- **Follow-up**: Informs the care team of the situation, suggests psychologist intervention.

- Respect for patient dignity and privacy

Respect for patient dignity and privacy is a fundamental value in the practice of internal medicine. It is the ethical foundation on which the relationship between caregiver and patient rests, and it is essential for preserving the patient's physical and psychological integrity. As a front-line healthcare professional, the nursing auxiliary plays a crucial role in implementing this principle on a daily basis. This chapter explores the dimensions of respect for dignity and privacy, the challenges encountered in the hospital environment, and strategies for integrating them fully into professional practice.

Understanding patient dignity and privacy

Dignity is a concept intrinsic to every human being, reflecting his or her worth, self-respect and right to be treated with consideration. Privacy, meanwhile, encompasses every individual's right to confidentiality, respect for their body and protection of their personal information. In the hospital environment, these notions take on particular importance, as patients are often in vulnerable situations, dependent on caregivers for their basic needs.

Ethical and legal foundations

Respect for dignity and privacy is governed by ethical principles and legislation. The Charter for hospitalized patients, for example, stipulates that "everyone is treated with respect. Their beliefs are respected. Their privacy and tranquillity are preserved". In addition, the Code of Ethics for the Health Professions insists on professional secrecy, informed consent and respect for patient rights.

These principles are not only legal obligations, but also moral commitments that reflect the humanism and caring inherent in the nursing profession. They guide the caregiver in his or her daily actions, ensuring that each patient is treated as a whole person, with his or her own needs, values and preferences.

Practices to respect patient dignity and privacy

1. **Ensuring the confidentiality of information**

   ◦ **Discretion in exchanges**: When conversing with patients, caregivers must be careful not to divulge sensitive information in the presence of other patients or the public. Discussions about the patient's state of health must take place in a private environment.

   ◦ **Protecting documents** : Medical records, care notes and personal information must be kept in a safe place. Caregivers must ensure that documents are not left in plain sight, and are accessible only to authorized persons.

2. Preserving physical privacy

○ **Respect during body care**: During hygiene care, it is essential to protect the patient's nudity as much as possible. Using sheets or towels to cover untreated parts of the body, closing curtains or doors, and informing the patient of forthcoming actions all contribute to preserving his or her privacy.

○ **Asking for consent**: Before carrying out any care or examination requiring physical contact, the caregiver must explain the procedure and obtain the patient's consent. This reinforces the patient's sense of control over his or her own body.

3. Respecting preferences and beliefs

○ **Personalizing care**: Adapting care to the patient's preferences in terms of modesty, culture or religion. For example, some patients may prefer to be cared for by a professional of the same sex.

○ **Diet and rituals**: Take into account specific dietary requirements, religious practices or spiritual needs, in collaboration with the care team.

4. Maintaining dignity in delicate situations

○ **Incontinence management**: Handle incontinence situations tactfully and promptly, without judgment or embarrassment for the patient. Ensure impeccable hygiene and total discretion.

○ **Respectful communication**: Use appropriate language, avoiding diminutives or infantilizing terms. Address patients by their surname, unless they prefer their first name, and be polite unless they wish to be addressed informally.

5. Promoting autonomy and participation

- **Encouraging independence**: Whenever possible, allow patients to carry out certain tasks themselves, such as dressing or feeding themselves. This boosts self-confidence and preserves dignity.

- **Involving the patient in decision-making**: Informing the patient about his or her state of health and planned care, and respecting his or her choices and refusals. Caregivers must support patients in their right to take charge of their own health.

6. Managing family visits and relationships

- **Respect for privacy**: During visits, ensure that the patient can receive his or her loved ones in an environment conducive to privacy. If care is to be provided, ask the patient whether he or she wishes visitors to remain present or not.

- **Confidentiality with relatives**: Only disclose medical information to family members with the patient's consent, in compliance with professional secrecy.

Challenges in the hospital environment

Respect for dignity and privacy can be put to the test by institutional constraints, such as staff shortages, overcrowding in shared rooms or the urgency of clinical situations. In such cases, the nursing auxiliary must show creativity and sensitivity to reconcile the demands of the service with respect for the patient.

- **Double or multiple rooms**: Use room dividers, lower your voice when talking, and be attentive to patient interactions to prevent discomfort.

- **Emergency situations**: Even in emergencies, strive to preserve the patient's privacy as far as possible, by explaining procedures and avoiding unnecessary exposure.

The impact of respect for dignity and privacy on the patient

Respecting patients' dignity and privacy has a positive impact on their well-being:

- **Reduced anxiety and stress**: Feeling respected and protected reduces anxiety linked to hospitalization and fosters a climate of trust.

- **Enhanced self-esteem**: Maintaining patients' dignity strengthens their sense of self-worth and autonomy.

- **Better collaboration in care**: A respected patient is more likely to participate actively in his or her care, to communicate openly and to follow medical recommendations.

- **Increased satisfaction**: Respect for dignity and privacy is a key indicator of the quality of care perceived by patients.

The caregiver's interpersonal skills

To ensure that dignity and privacy are respected, the caregiver must develop certain interpersonal skills:

- **Empathy**: Putting yourself in the patient's shoes, understanding their emotions and needs.

- **Assertive communication**: Expressing information clearly and respectfully, while listening to the patient's reactions.

- **Discretion**: Keep sensitive information to yourself, avoid inappropriate discussions in the presence of others.

- **Observation**: Detect signs of discomfort, discomfort or discomfort in the patient, and adapt your approach accordingly.

Ongoing training and awareness-raising

Ongoing training is essential to maintain a high level of competence in respecting dignity and privacy:

- **Workshops and seminars**: Participate in training courses on ethics, communication and managing delicate situations.

- **Supervision and exchanges**: Discuss challenges encountered with colleagues and superiors, share best practices.

- **Self-evaluation**: Reflect on your own practice, identify areas for improvement, be open to constructive feedback.

Case studies to illustrate the principles

1. **Hygiene care for a modest patient**
   Mr Dupont, aged 65, needs to be fully groomed in bed. He expresses discomfort at the idea of being naked in front of the nursing staff.

   - **The caregiver's approach**: Before starting, the caregiver calmly explains the procedure, reassures Mr. Dupont that his privacy will be respected, and suggests that he cover any unwashed areas with a towel. He closes the door and draws the curtains to ensure confidentiality.

2. **Confidential discussion in a shared room**

   Mrs. Martin wishes to discuss her concerns about her diagnosis, but she shares her room with another patient.

   ◦ **Solution**: The caregiver suggests that Mrs. Martin accompany her to a more private area, such as a consulting room or a quiet corner of the ward, where she can talk freely.

- Managing difficult or end-of-life patients

Managing difficult or end-of-life patients represents a major challenge for Internal Medicine healthcare professionals. These situations require not only technical skills, but also great sensitivity, empathy and the ability to communicate effectively. The caregiver, by virtue of his or her proximity to the patient, plays a crucial role in providing accompaniment and support, helping to improve the quality of care and the patient's well-being. This chapter explores strategies and approaches for managing these complex situations with professionalism and humanity.

Understanding difficult patients

Difficult patients may display aggressive, hostile, anxious or uncooperative behaviours. These attitudes may be the result of various factors:

- **Pain or physical discomfort**: Suffering can lead to irritability or agitation.
- **Anxiety and fear**: Fear of illness, medical procedures or the unknown can provoke defensive reactions.
- **Psychiatric disorders**: pathologies such as depression, schizophrenia or bipolar disorder can influence behavior.
- **Personal history**: Previous negative experiences with the healthcare system can affect patient confidence.
- **Social or family isolation**: Lack of support can exacerbate feelings of vulnerability.

Approaches to managing difficult patients

1. **Maintain a calm, professional attitude**

   ○ **Controlling your own emotions**: Remaining calm in the face of a patient's aggressiveness or frustration prevents the situation from escalating.
   ○ **Use a soothing tone of voice**: Speak softly and clearly to reassure the patient.
   ○ **Adopt an open posture**: show availability and active listening without judgment.

2. **Establishing effective communication**

   ○ **Active listening**: Allowing patients to express their concerns without interruption, while showing empathy.
   ○ **Clarify misunderstandings**: Check mutual understanding, rephrase what the patient has said to make sure they feel heard.
   ○ **Provide clear information**: Explain procedures, treatments and reasons for care in an understandable way.

3. **Acknowledging and validating the patient's feelings**

   ○ **Empathy**: Acknowledging the patient's distress by saying, for example, "I understand how difficult this situation is for you".
   ○ **Avoid confrontation**: Don't contradict or minimize the patient's feelings, even if they seem disproportionate.

4. **Involving the patient in care**

   ○ **Encouraging autonomy**: Allowing patients to participate in decisions concerning their care reinforces their sense of control.

- ○ **Offer choices**: Provide options whenever possible, even for small decisions such as the order of care.

5. Working with the care team

- ○ **Sharing information**: Inform the team of difficulties encountered, triggers identified and effective strategies.
- ○ **Plan coordinated interventions**: Develop a personalized care plan to meet the patient's specific needs.
- ○ **Call on specialized professionals**: If necessary, seek the intervention of a psychologist, psychiatrist or mediator.

6. Ensure your own safety and that of others

- ○ **Respect safety protocols**: In the event of physical aggression, maintain a safe distance, have a clear exit.
- ○ **Ask for help**: Don't hesitate to call on colleagues or security if the situation calls for it.
- ○ **Crisis management training**: Participate in training courses on managing aggressive behavior.

Supporting patients at the end of life

Patients at the end of life require special attention, focused on symptom relief, emotional support and respect for their wishes. Caregivers play an essential role in this process.

Principles of palliative care

- • **Relieve pain and symptoms**: Work with the team to ensure optimal comfort, monitoring and reporting signs of pain, dyspnea or anxiety.

- **Respecting the patient's wishes**: knowing and respecting advance directives and wishes concerning care and the end of life.
- **Offer a comforting presence**: Being present, listening, gently touching can bring great comfort.

Approaches to supporting patients at the end of life

1. **Empathetic communication**

- ◦ **Attentive listening**: allowing patients to express their fears, regrets and hopes.
- ◦ **Verbal support**: Use encouraging phrases, avoid false hope and remain positive.
- ◦ **Respectful silence**: Sometimes shared silence is more meaningful than words.

2. **Spiritual and cultural support**

- ◦ **Respecting beliefs**: Facilitating access to spiritual or religious resources if the patient so wishes.
- ◦ **Integrate rituals**: Allow cultural or spiritual practices that bring comfort.

3. **Involving family and friends**

- ◦ **Facilitate visits**: Arrange schedules or space to enable loved ones to be present.
- ◦ **Supporting family members**: Listening to them, informing them of developments, guiding them in their role with the patient.
- ◦ **Encourage exchanges**: Encourage moments of intimacy for farewells or meaningful sharing.

4. Managing non-painful symptoms

- ○ **Physical comfort**: maintaining good hygiene, preventing bedsores, ensuring comfortable positioning.
- ○ **Sign monitoring**: Observe changes in the patient's condition to adjust care accordingly.

5. Respect for dignity

- ○ **Preserving privacy**: Continuing to respect the patient's body, even in the final moments.
- ○ **Valuing the person**: Recognizing his or her history, values and achievements.

6. Taking care of yourself as a caregiver

- ○ **Recognize your own emotions**: Accept that end-of-life care can be trying.
- ○ **Seek support**: Talk to colleagues, take part in discussion or supervision groups.
- ○ **Personal equilibrium**: Maintain relaxing activities outside work to preserve your well-being.

Specific challenges and adaptation strategies

- **Managing mental distress**: Some patients may express existential distress. Listening to and validating their feelings is crucial.
- **Patients with no family**: Offer an even stronger presence, working with volunteers or associations where possible.
- **Complex ethical situations**: Dealing with requests for euthanasia or refusal of care means referring to protocols and laws in force, and involving the multidisciplinary team.

Case study: Supporting a patient at the end of life

Mrs L., aged 78, is hospitalized with terminal heart failure. She expresses her fear of dying and her regret at not having seen her son again, with whom she is in conflict.

- **The caregiver's approach** :

  ◦ **Empathetic listening**: Let Mrs L. express her feelings, without judging or pressuring her.
  ◦ **Emotional support**: reassure her that it's normal to feel these emotions, offer comfort.
  ◦ **Offer of help**: Ask her if she would like the team to contact her son, respecting her decision.
  ◦ **Collaboration with the team**: Inform the referral nurse to consider psychological support.

Chapter 5

Emergency management

- Recognizing clinical warning signs

The ability to recognize clinical warning signs is an essential skill for the internal medicine orderly. This ability enables early detection of potential deterioration in a patient's state of health, promoting rapid intervention by the medical team. By being alert to subtle or abrupt changes in patients' clinical parameters and behavior, the orderly makes a significant contribution to preventing serious complications and improving prognosis.

The importance of clinical vigilance

Patients hospitalized in Internal Medicine often present with complex pathologies, and may be subject to rapid fluctuations in their state of health. Early recognition of warning signs is crucial to avoid worsening symptoms, cardiac arrest, septic shock or other critical situations. The caregiver, through his or her constant presence with patients, is in the front line to observe these signs and quickly alert the nursing team.

Warning signs to watch out for

1. **Changes in consciousness**

   A sudden change in level of consciousness is a major warning sign. This includes unusual drowsiness, confusion, agitation, impaired orientation or loss of consciousness. For example, a previously alert patient who suddenly becomes lethargic or unresponsive to verbal stimuli requires immediate attention.

2. **Vital sign abnormalities**

   - **Heart rate**: Tachycardia (heart rate above 100 beats per minute) or bradycardia (below 60 beats per minute) may indicate a heart problem, bleeding or drug reaction.
   - **Blood pressure**: Hypotension (low blood pressure) can signal shock, dehydration or hemorrhage. Severe hypertension can lead to cardiovascular or neurological complications.

- **Respiratory rate**: Tachypnea (rapid breathing) or bradypnea (slow breathing) may indicate respiratory distress, metabolic acidosis or intoxication.
- **Oxygen saturation**: A drop in oxygen saturation below 90% is cause for concern and requires intervention to prevent tissue hypoxia.
- **Body temperature**: A high fever may indicate a severe infection, while hypothermia may indicate shock or prolonged exposure to cold.

3. Sudden, intense pain

The onset of acute pain, especially if localized in the chest, abdomen or head, should be taken seriously. For example, constrictive chest pain may be a sign of myocardial infarction, requiring urgent treatment.

4. Signs of respiratory distress

Breathing difficulties, dyspnea, wheezing, cyanosis (bluish coloration of the lips or extremities) or use of accessory muscles for breathing are indicators of possible respiratory failure or airway obstruction.

5. Neurological changes

The sudden onset of muscle weakness, paralysis, slurred speech, convulsions or loss of feeling may indicate a stroke or epileptic seizure.

6. Abnormalities in urine or stool

Urinary retention, anuria (absence of urine), blood in the urine (hematuria) or stools (melena) are important warning signs. Similarly, severe diarrhea can lead to rapid dehydration.

7. Disturbing skin signs

The appearance of sudden skin rashes, urticaria, extensive redness or angioedema (swelling of the face, lips and tongue) may signal a serious allergic reaction, such as anaphylactic shock.

8. **Signs of bleeding**
   Any heavy bleeding, whether external or internal (hematemesis, rectal bleeding), should be treated as an emergency. Spontaneous bruising or petechiae may indicate coagulation disorders.

9. **Changes in general condition**
   Extreme fatigue, marked pallor, cold sweats, unexplained malaise or a "bad feeling" expressed by the patient are signals not to be overlooked.

10. **Behavioral changes**
   Psychomotor agitation, hallucinations, unusual or aggressive behavior may be signs of delirium, hypoglycemia or encephalopathy.

The active role of the caregiver

The caregiver must adopt a proactive attitude to detect these warning signs:

- **Continuous observation**: Take advantage of daily interactions (toilets, meals, mobilizations) to assess the patient's condition.
- **Attentive listening**: Take into account the patient's complaints, even if they seem harmless. Sometimes, a simple "I don't feel well" can precede clinical deterioration.
- **Regular measurement of parameters**: Take vital signs according to protocols, and repeat measurements in the event of anomalies.
- **Rigorous documentation**: Make a precise note of observations in the patient record, indicating the time and exact values.

- **Immediate communication**: Report any abnormality to the nurse or doctor without delay. It's better to alert to a false alarm than to miss a critical sign.

Collaboration with the care team

Effective communication with the team is essential:

- **Clear verbal communication**: During team changes, share relevant information, emphasizing observed warning signs.
- **Participation in meetings**: Contribute to discussions on patients' condition, provide concrete observations.
- **Compliance with emergency protocols**: Know the procedures to follow in critical situations (call the doctor, set up first aid).

Training and updating knowledge

To be effective in recognizing warning signs, the caregiver must :

- **Regular training**: Participate in training courses on emergencies, common internal medicine pathologies and first aid.
- **Update your knowledge**: Keep abreast of new recommendations, institutional protocols and medical advances.
- **Self-evaluation**: Reflect on your practice, identify areas for improvement, seek feedback from the team.

Special cases

- **Elderly patients**: Warning signs may be atypical in the elderly. Sudden confusion may be the only sign of infection or infarction.
- **Non-communicative patients**: In aphasic or unconscious patients, observation of non-verbal signs (facial

expressions, movements, physiological reactions) is essential.

- **Patients with cognitive impairment**: Patients with dementia may have difficulty expressing their symptoms. Changes in behavior or appetite may indicate a medical problem.

The importance of responsiveness

Quick action can save lives. The orderly must :

- **Don't hesitate**: When in doubt, always report an anomaly.
- **Follow protocols**: apply emergency procedures, ensure patient safety (lateral position, oxygen administration if authorized).
- **Remaining calm**: Keeping your cool to act effectively, reassuring the patient and family.

- Emergency protocols and internal procedures

Mastery of emergency protocols and internal procedures is a crucial skill for the internal medicine orderly. In an environment where patients often present with complex pathologies, and where situations can evolve rapidly, precise knowledge of these protocols enables them to respond effectively to emergencies, guarantee patient safety and contribute to the smooth running of the department. This chapter explores the importance of these protocols, the main types of emergencies encountered, and the specific roles of the nursing auxiliary in implementing them.

The importance of emergency protocols and internal procedures

Emergency protocols are pre-established guidelines describing the actions to be taken in critical situations. They aim to standardize responses, reduce errors and ensure rapid, coordinated care.

Internal procedures, on the other hand, provide a framework for day-to-day practices, individual responsibilities and administrative processes within the healthcare facility.

For the nursing auxiliary, knowledge of these protocols is essential for several reasons:

- **Reactivity to emergencies**: Be able to identify an emergency situation and take appropriate action without delay.
- **Patient safety**: Ensuring that procedures performed comply with best practices and institutional standards.
- **Effective collaboration**: Facilitate communication and coordination with the care team using a common language and shared procedures.
- **Professional responsibility**: Respect legal and ethical obligations, acting within the framework defined by the establishment.

Main types of internal medicine emergencies

1. Cardiopulmonary arrest (CPR)

- ○ **Recognition**: Absence of consciousness, normal breathing and palpable pulse.
- ○ **Immediate action**:
  - ▪ **Alert**: Immediately call the resuscitation team or activate the internal alert system (code blue).
  - ▪ **Cardiopulmonary resuscitation (CPR)**: Start chest compressions according to current protocols, while waiting for the specialized team to arrive.
  - ▪ **Use of automated external defibrillator (AED)**: If available and trained in its use, follow the device's instructions.

- Role of the orderly : Ensure the safety of the scene, perform basic CPR, help set up equipment, support the team during the intervention.

2. Acute respiratory distress

- **Clinical signs**: Severe dyspnea, cyanosis, tachypnea, use of accessory muscles, low oxygen saturation.
- **Immediate action**:
  - **Patient positioning**: Place the patient in a seated or semi-seated position to facilitate breathing.
  - **Administer oxygen**: If authorized and prescribed, set up appropriate oxygen therapy.
  - **Alert the medical team**: quickly inform the nurse and doctor.
- **Role of the caregiver** : Monitor vital signs, reassure the patient, prepare equipment for the team (nebulizer, suction).

3. Severe hypoglycemia

- **Clinical signs**: Confusion, sweating, tremors, convulsions, loss of consciousness.
- **Immediate action**:
  - **Measuring capillary blood glucose**: Confirming the diagnosis.
  - **Administer sugar**: If the patient is conscious, give a sugary drink or glucose tablets.
  - **In case of unconsciousness**: do not give anything by mouth, place the patient in the lateral safety position.
  - **Alert**: Inform the nurse for urgent medical care.

- ○ **Role of the caregiver**: Monitor the patient, prevent complications, prepare equipment for glucagon injections.

4. Acute allergic reaction (anaphylaxis)

- ○ **Clinical signs**: rash, angioedema, breathing difficulties, hypotension, tachycardia.
- ○ **Immediate action**:
  - ▪ **Interrupt exposure to allergen**: Stop any suspected infusion.
  - ▪ **Alert immediately**: Notify the medical team.
  - ▪ **Position the patient**: Lie with legs elevated if hypotension, or semi-seated position if dyspnea.
- ○ **Role of the caregiver** : Monitor vital signs, prepare emergency equipment (adrenaline, oxygen), reassure the patient.

5. Fall or trauma

- ○ **Immediate action**:
  - ▪ **Assess patient's condition**: Check for consciousness, apparent injuries.
  - ▪ **Do not mobilize the patient unnecessarily**: If trauma is suspected, avoid movement.
  - ▪ **Alert**: Inform the nurse and doctor.
- ○ **Caregiver's role**: Protect the patient, apply first aid if necessary, document the incident according to internal procedures.

Internal procedures and the caregiver's role

1. Reporting adverse events

- ○ **Importance**: Helps improve quality of care and prevent incidents from recurring.
- ○ **Procedure**:
  - ▪ **Document the event**: Precise description of facts, time, witnesses.
  - ▪ **Use specific forms**: According to facility guidelines.
  - ▪ **Pass on to management**: Inform the health executive or quality consultant.
- ○ **Role of the caregiver**: Be vigilant and report any incident, however minor.

2. Managing nosocomial infections

- ○ **Application of hygiene protocols**: hand washing, use of personal protective equipment, compliance with standard and additional precautions.
- ○ **Monitoring at-risk patients**: Identify signs of infection, observe isolation measures.
- ○ **Participation in training courses**: Keep abreast of protocol updates.
- ○ **The role of the nursing auxiliary** : Play an active role in infection prevention, raising awareness among patients and visitors.

3. Medication management

- ○ **Compliance with drug circuits**: storage, preparation, administration (according to assigned role).
- ○ **Check expiration dates**: Regularly check medicines and medical devices.
- ○ **Securing stocks**: Ensure that medicines are stored in appropriate conditions.

- **Role of the orderly** : Help prepare care carts, report any anomalies, comply with traceability rules.

4. Evacuation in the event of a major emergency

- **Knowledge of evacuation plan**: location of emergency exits, fire extinguishers, assembly points.
- **Participate in drills**: Train regularly to be ready in the event of a real disaster.
- **Patient assistance**: Help evacuate patients, respecting priorities and safety instructions.
- **Caregiver's role**: Act calmly and efficiently, coordinate with the team, ensure the safety of vulnerable patients.

Training and updating knowledge

Mastering emergency protocols and internal procedures requires ongoing training:

- **Participate in training sessions**: mandatory or optional, organized by the company.
- **Become familiar with written protocols**: Regularly read documents, posters and manuals.
- **Simulations and practical exercises**: Take part in role-playing exercises to reinforce skills.
- **Team discussions**: Discuss concrete cases, feedback and possible improvements.

Legal and ethical responsibilities

Caregivers are required to follow protocols for :

- **Ensuring safe care**: avoiding errors that could endanger the patient.
- **Protect professional liability**: In the event of an incident, demonstrate compliance with procedures.

- **Contribute to service quality**: Participate in the continuous improvement of practices.

Collaboration with the multidisciplinary team

- **Effective communication**: convey information clearly and precisely, use appropriate vocabulary.
- **Respecting roles**: knowing the limits of your competencies, knowing when and to whom to delegate or refer.
- **Team spirit**: work in synergy with nurses, doctors and other professionals.

Case studies to illustrate protocols

1. **Sudden hypotension in a patient**

   - **Observation**: The patient presents with dizziness, pallor and cold sweat.
   - **Actions of the caregiver** :
     - Lay patient supine, elevate legs.
     - Measure blood pressure and record values.
     - Alert the nurse immediately.
     - Stay with the patient to reassure him/her and monitor progress.

2. **Detecting a medication error**

   - **Situation**: A drug intended for another patient was inadvertently placed on the bedside table.
   - **Actions of the caregiver** :
     - Remove drug immediately.
     - Inform the nurse or health executive.

- Document the incident according to internal procedure.
- Participate in the analysis of the event to avoid its repetition.

- The caregiver's role in critical interventions

In the demanding field of internal medicine, critical interventions are emergency situations requiring a rapid, coordinated and effective response from the nursing team. Although often perceived as a secondary player, the nursing auxiliary plays an essential role in these decisive moments. Their knowledge of protocols, proximity to patients and ability to act under pressure make them an indispensable link in the care chain. This chapter explores in depth the role of the caregiver during critical interventions, highlighting his or her responsibilities, specific skills and the impact of his or her action on the patient's prognosis.

Understanding critical interventions

Critical interventions encompass all situations where the patient's life is in immediate danger and rapid care is crucial. This includes cardiorespiratory arrest, hemorrhagic shock, acute respiratory distress, anaphylactic reactions, stroke, severe epileptic seizures, and many other medical emergencies. These situations require immediate mobilization of the care team, effective communication and rigorous application of emergency protocols.

Preparation and daily vigilance

The caregiver's role in critical interventions begins long before the emergency occurs. Their day-to-day vigilance, in-depth knowledge of patients and ability to recognize warning signs can often prevent critical situations from arising, or enable them to react more quickly.

- **Careful monitoring**: By being in constant contact with patients, the caregiver observes subtle changes in their state of health. Changes in consciousness, abnormal vital signs, unexplained agitation or unusual complaints can be the first signs of rapid deterioration.

- **Background knowledge**: Understanding the specific pathologies and risks of each patient enables the caregiver to anticipate possible complications. For example, a cardiac patient with chest pains requires immediate attention.

- **Mastery of protocols**: Familiarity with emergency procedures and internal protocols ensures an appropriate response in the event of a crisis. Caregivers must be regularly trained in first aid, cardiopulmonary resuscitation (CPR) and the use of emergency equipment.

Immediate action in the event of a critical intervention

When a critical situation arises, the caregiver intervenes proactively and in coordination with the nursing team. Their immediate actions can make the difference between life and death.

1. Detection and warning

- **Emergency recognition**: Quickly identify the seriousness of the situation, whether it's loss of consciousness, lack of breathing, massive bleeding or any other critical sign.

- **Alerting the team**: Use the appropriate means of communication to immediately inform the nurse in charge and the doctor. In some facilities, this may involve activating a specific emergency code (e.g. code blue for cardiorespiratory arrest).

2. First aid

- ○ **Basic resuscitation**: If trained and authorized, the caregiver can start CPR while waiting for the medical team to arrive. This includes chest compressions and, if possible, mouth-to-mouth resuscitation or the use of an automated external defibrillator (AED).

- ○ **Vital assistance**: Clear the airway, place the patient in the lateral safety position in the event of convulsions or vomiting, control external bleeding by direct compression.

- ○ **Securing the environment**: ensuring the patient is in an accessible area, clearing obstacles, preventing falls or further injury.

3. Medical team support

- ○ **Material preparation**: Bring in the emergency cart, prepare the necessary equipment (oxygen, infusion equipment, emergency medication).

- ○ **Active collaboration**: Follow the nurse's and doctor's instructions, assist with advanced resuscitation maneuvers, provide relevant patient information (history, previous emergency events).

- ○ **Environmental management**: Remove other patients or visitors to ensure the privacy of the patient in distress, while maintaining an environment conducive to intervention.

Psychological support and communication

In addition to technical care, the caregiver provides essential psychological support, both to the patient and to the family members present.

- **Reassure the patient**: If the patient is conscious, talk to him calmly, explain what's happening and encourage him to remain calm.

- **Dealing with relatives**: Informing family members in an empathetic way, inviting them to wait in an appropriate place, while respecting confidentiality protocols.

- **Communicating with the team**: Clearly communicating information, reporting any changes in the patient's condition, acting as an effective relay between the various parties involved.

After the critical intervention

Once the situation has stabilized, the caregiver's role continues with monitoring and continuity of care.

- **Close monitoring**: Continue to observe patient for recurrence or complications, measure vital signs as directed.

- **Documentation**: Participate in the drafting of incident reports, noting actions taken, schedules, relevant observations.

- **Moral support**: Being there for the patient who may be distressed by the event, offering an attentive ear, facilitating communication with the medical team.

- **Debriefing**: Participate in team meetings to analyze the intervention, identify strengths and areas for improvement, and contribute to collective learning.

Further training and preparation

The nursing auxiliary's competence in critical interventions is based on sound training and regular updating of knowledge.

- **Specific training**: Participate in training courses in cardiopulmonary resuscitation, emergency management, use of emergency equipment.

- **Simulations**: Take part in practical exercises and scenarios to reinforce reflexes and team coordination.

- **Knowledge of protocols**: Keep abreast of internal protocol updates and new medical recommendations.

Ethics and responsibilities

During critical interventions, the nursing auxiliary must act in accordance with ethical principles and the limits of its function.

- **Respecting competencies**: Intervene within the scope of its remit, without encroaching on procedures reserved for nurses or doctors, except in cases of vital necessity and within the limits of acquired competencies.

- **Confidentiality**: Protect patient information from unauthorized disclosure, even in stressful situations.

- **Professionalism**: Maintain a calm demeanor, keep emotions in check, exercise discernment and composure.

Impact on patient and team

The caregiver's role in critical interventions has a significant impact on the patient and on team dynamics.

- **For the patient**: Rapid, appropriate intervention increases the chances of survival, reduces the risk of after-effects and contributes to recovery.

- **For the team**: The orderly facilitates the work of nurses and doctors, promotes coordinated intervention, and strengthens cohesion and collective efficiency.

- **For the caregiver**: These experiences, while stressful, are also rewarding. They develop skills, boost confidence and reinforce a sense of professional accomplishment.

Challenges and stress management

Critical interventions can be a source of intense stress for the caregiver.

- **Stress management**: Learn to manage your emotions, use breathing techniques, prepare yourself mentally for emergency situations.

- **Team support**: Don't hesitate to share your feelings with colleagues, and take part in psychological debriefings if necessary.

- **Personal balance**: look after your well-being outside work, take part in relaxing activities, maintain a healthy lifestyle.

- Stress management in emergency situations

The ability to manage stress in emergency situations is an essential skill for the internal medicine orderly. Medical emergencies are moments of intense tension when every second counts, and when the quality of the response can have a direct impact on the patient's life. If left unchecked, stress can impair performance, decision-making and communication, compromising the effectiveness of the response. This chapter explores the mechanisms of stress in the emergency context, strategies for managing it effectively, and the importance of this skill for professional well-being and quality of care.

Understanding stress in emergency situations

Stress is a normal physiological and psychological reaction to threat or pressure. In emergency situations, the body triggers a "fight or flight" response, releasing hormones such as adrenalin and cortisol. These substances prepare the body to react quickly, increasing alertness, heart rate and muscle tension. However, excessive or poorly managed stress can have negative effects:

- **Impaired cognitive functions**: difficulty concentrating, memory impairment, impulsive decision-making.
- **Intense emotional reactions**: anxiety, irritability, feelings of helplessness.
- **Physical manifestations**: Tremors, sweating, palpitations, digestive disorders.

Understanding these mechanisms enables caregivers to recognize their own reactions to stress and implement strategies to manage them.

The importance of preparation and training

Proper preparation is the first step towards effective stress management. Confidence in one's skills and familiarity with emergency procedures reduce anxiety and improve performance.

- **Ongoing training**: Regularly attend training courses on emergency protocols, cardiopulmonary resuscitation and the use of emergency equipment.
- **Practical simulations**: Take part in role-playing exercises to reinforce reflexes, team coordination and self-confidence.
- **Knowledge of protocols**: Keep abreast of updates to internal procedures, evacuation plans and emergency numbers.

Pre-emergency stress management techniques

- **Mental preparation**: visualize possible emergency situations, anticipate actions to be taken, mentally familiarize yourself with procedures.
- **Lifestyle**: Maintain a balanced diet, sufficient sleep and regular physical activity to boost resistance to stress.
- **Relaxation and meditation**: Practice relaxation, deep breathing or meditation techniques to reduce overall stress levels.

Emergency stress management

1. **Breathing control**

   Breathing is a powerful tool for managing stress in real time. In emergency situations :

   - **Deep breathing**: Inhale slowly through the nose, exhale through the mouth, helping to reduce heart rate and muscle tension.
   - **Cardiac coherence**: adopt a regular breathing rhythm to stabilize emotions and improve mental clarity.

2. **Focus on the task**

   - **Focus on the present**: concentrate on the immediate actions to be taken, without being distracted by potential consequences.
   - **Breaking down actions**: Break down complex tasks into simple steps to avoid overwhelm.

3. **Effective communication**

   - **Use of clear language**: Express yourself concisely with the team, using standardized communication codes or protocols.

o   **Active listening**: pay attention to colleagues' instructions, check mutual understanding.

4.   Emotional control

o   **Self-observation**: Recognize your own emotions without letting them interfere with action.
o   **Managing negative thoughts**: Replace catastrophic thoughts with positive or neutral affirmations.

Team role and mutual support

Teamwork is essential for managing stress in emergency situations. A good group dynamic promotes trust, coordination and efficiency.

- **Team cohesion**: Developing solid professional relationships based on respect and trust.
- **Mutual support**: Be alert to signs of stress in colleagues, offer help or encouragement.
- **Shared leadership**: Recognize each other's skills, accept direction from colleagues where appropriate.

After the emergency: debriefing and recovery

Stress management doesn't stop once the emergency is over. It's important to take time to decompress and learn from the experience.

1.   Operational debriefing

o   **Analysis of the intervention**: Bring the team together to discuss what went well, any difficulties encountered and areas for improvement.

- ○ **Expression of feelings**: Enable everyone to share their emotions and impressions in a caring environment.

2. Managing post-event stress

- ○ **Rest and recuperation**: Take the time to rest physically and mentally after a stressful operation.
- ○ **Relaxing activities**: Take part in leisure activities that promote relaxation, such as reading, music and gentle exercise.
- ○ **Psychological support**: If necessary, consult a professional to manage the effects of traumatic stress.

Building long-term resilience

Resilience is the ability to adapt and bounce back from difficult situations. To reinforce this quality :

- **Continuous learning**: See every situation as an opportunity for learning and development.
- **Adaptability**: Cultivate mental flexibility to adjust to the unexpected.
- **Positive attitude**: Maintain an optimistic outlook, focusing on success and progress.

Taking care of yourself to better care for others

The caregiver's mental and physical health is fundamental to providing quality care. Taking care of oneself is a professional responsibility.

- **Professional limits**: Recognize your limits, know how to say no when the load is too heavy.
- **Work/life balance**: Making time for personal activities and socializing outside work.

- **Wellness training**: Participate in workshops or training courses on stress management and burn-out prevention.

Case study: Real-life application

During a night shift, a patient suddenly presents with acute respiratory distress. The orderly, initially taken by surprise, applies stress management techniques:

- **Deep breathing**: He takes a deep breath to calm his nervousness.
- **Focus on action**: He concentrates on the steps to follow: alert the team, place the patient in a semi-seated position, prepare the oxygen.
- **Clear communication**: informs the nurse of the situation with precise information.
- **Patient support**: reassures the patient, explains what's happening, encourages calm breathing.
- **After the intervention**: He takes part in the debriefing with the team, expresses his emotions and listens to feedback.

This approach enables him to manage the situation effectively, maintain his composure and make a positive contribution to the patient's care.

Chapter 6

Professional ethics and deontology

- Confidentiality and medical secrecy

Confidentiality and medical secrecy are fundamental principles of care in internal medicine. They are the ethical and legal pillars that protect patient privacy and preserve the essential trust between patients and healthcare professionals. For the caregiver, respecting these principles is a major responsibility that guides every interaction with the patient, every exchange of information and every act of care. This chapter explores in depth the notions of confidentiality and medical secrecy, their importance in daily practice, the associated legal obligations and the challenges caregivers may face.

Understanding medical confidentiality

Medical confidentiality is the legal and moral obligation for all healthcare professionals not to divulge personal health information concerning a patient. It is enshrined in the French Public Health Code (Code de la santé publique) and the French Criminal Code (Code pénal), and its violation may result in criminal, civil and disciplinary sanctions.

Medical confidentiality covers all information relating to a patient's health, gathered directly or indirectly in the course of professional practice. This includes diagnoses, treatments, medical history and test results, as well as personal confidences, lifestyle habits and family or social information.

Ethical and legal foundations

1. Professional ethics

- **Respect for the individual**: Medical confidentiality is an expression of respect for patient autonomy and dignity. It guarantees that sensitive information is protected, enabling patients to confide in us without fear of disclosure.

- **Therapeutic trust**: A relationship of trust between patient and caregiver is essential for effective care.

122

Respecting medical confidentiality reinforces this trust, encouraging patients to share information that is crucial to their health.

2. Legal framework

- ○ **Public Health Code (Article L.1110-4)**: It stipulates that "any person under the care of a healthcare professional [...] has the right to respect for his or her private life and the secrecy of information concerning him or her".

- ○ **Penal Code (Article 226-13)**: Violation of professional secrecy is punishable by one year's imprisonment and a fine of 15,000 euros.

- ○ **Legal exceptions**: In certain specific situations, medical secrecy may be lifted, notably in the case of mandatory reporting of certain infectious diseases, abuse of minors or vulnerable persons, or at the request of the courts. However, these exceptions are strictly regulated by law.

The caregiver's role in respecting medical confidentiality

1. Information access

- ○ **Necessary information**: Caregivers have access to the information they need to carry out their duties. He/she must use it only in the context of patient care.

- ○ **Limiting access**: He must not seek to obtain information that is not relevant to his role or that has not been communicated to him in a professional context.

2. Communication with the care team

- **Limited sharing**: Patient medical information may be shared with members of the healthcare team involved in the patient's care, in compliance with "shared confidentiality".

- **Professional discretion**: Discussions concerning patients should take place in appropriate places, away from uninvolved third parties (other patients, visitors, non-medical staff).

3. Patient interaction

- **Respect for privacy**: During care, the caregiver must ensure the confidentiality of exchanges, making sure that conversations are not overheard by others.

- **Answering questions**: If a patient asks questions about his/her state of health or specific medical information, the caregiver must answer within the limits of his/her competence and, if necessary, refer the patient to the nurse or doctor.

4. Relations with relatives

- **Patient consent**: Medical information should only be communicated to relatives if the patient has given explicit consent, except in the case of incapacity or a special situation provided for by law.

- **Handling requests**: In the event of a request for information from relatives, the caregiver must respect medical confidentiality and, if necessary, refer them to the doctor or health executive.

Special situations and challenges

1. Informal conversations

- **Avoid inappropriate discussions**: Discussions about patients in public areas of the hospital (corridors, elevators, cafeteria) or outside the professional environment should be avoided.

- **Social networks**: The publication of photos, comments or information about patients on social networks is strictly forbidden and constitutes a breach of professional secrecy.

2. Patient confessions

- **Handling sensitive information**: Patients may entrust caregivers with personal or family information. Such confidences must be treated with the utmost discretion.

- **Referral to professionals**: If the patient raises concerns (abuse, psychological distress), the caregiver must inform the care team, in accordance with internal procedures, without betraying the patient's trust.

3. Exceptions to medical confidentiality

- **Legal obligation**: In certain situations, such as the endangerment of others, abuse of minors or vulnerable persons, the caregiver is obliged to report the facts to the competent authorities.

- **Procedure to be followed**: These situations must be managed in collaboration with the medical team and the health executive, in compliance with institutional protocols.

Strategies for preserving confidentiality

1. Working environment

- ◦ **Private areas**: Use treatment rooms or offices for confidential discussions, close doors, make sure no one is listening in.

- ◦ **Medical documents**: Keep patient files in secure locations, and do not leave documents containing personal information lying around.

2. Written and electronic communication

- ◦ **E-mails and messages**: Use secure channels to send medical information, avoid communications on non-secure platforms.

- ◦ **Traceability**: Ensure that notes in the patient file are factual, relevant and professionally written.

3. Training and awareness-raising

- ◦ **Regular updates**: Participate in training courses on medical secrecy, new regulations and best practices in confidentiality.

- ◦ **Sharing experiences**: Discuss complex situations and ethical dilemmas with colleagues, to reinforce collective understanding.

The consequences of breaching medical confidentiality

1. Legal penalties

- ◦ **Penalties**: One year's imprisonment and a 15,000-euro fine, in accordance with article 226-13 of the French Penal Code.

- **Civil**: Repair of damage caused to the patient, compensation.

- **Disciplinary**: professional sanctions up to and including dismissal.

2. Damage to the relationship of trust

- **Loss of trust**: Breach of medical confidentiality can break down the relationship of trust with the patient, adversely affecting his or her care and well-being.

- **Impact on the establishment**: The hospital's reputation may be affected, leading to a loss of credibility and public confidence.

Concrete examples to illustrate the principles

1. Request for information from a relative
A member of Mr. Dupont's family asks the caregiver for details about his state of health.

- **Appropriate response**: "I understand your concern for Mr. Dupont. I suggest you discuss this with the doctor or nurse, who will be able to give you the necessary information."

2. Conversation in public spaces
Two orderlies discuss a patient's care in the corridor.

- **Best practice**: Avoid mentioning identifiable information, postpone the conversation to a private place, be aware of who is nearby.

- Patient rights and informed consent

Recognition and respect for patients' rights are fundamental principles guiding the practice of internal medicine. Informed consent, in particular, lies at the heart of the relationship between caregiver and patient, reflecting respect for the autonomy, dignity and freedom of each individual. The caregiver, as an essential member of the care team, has a key role to play in promoting and protecting these rights. This chapter explores the concepts of patient rights and informed consent, their importance in daily practice, the associated legal and ethical obligations, and the challenges encountered in implementing them.

Understanding patient rights

Patient rights are legal and ethical guarantees designed to protect people receiving healthcare. They include the right to information, the right to free and informed consent, the right to privacy and confidentiality, the right to dignity, the right to refuse treatment and the right to access one's medical records.

Fundamental principles of patient rights

1. **Right to information**
   Patients have the right to receive clear, comprehensible and appropriate information on their state of health, the examinations and treatments proposed, their benefits, risks and alternatives. This information must enable them to make informed decisions about their health.

2. **Free and informed consent**
   Before any medical procedure or treatment, patients must give their free and informed consent, i.e. without pressure or coercion, after receiving all the necessary information.

3. **Right to privacy and confidentiality**
   Patients' personal and medical information must be protected, and professional secrecy must be respected by all healthcare professionals.

4. **Right to dignity and respect**
   Patients must be treated with respect, courtesy and consideration, without discrimination.

5. **Right to refuse or discontinue treatment**
   Patients have the right to refuse treatment, even if this could have serious consequences for their health, provided they are fully informed of the implications.

6. **Right to access medical records**
   Patients have the right to consult and obtain a copy of their medical record, to better understand their health or to share it with another healthcare professional.

The caregiver's role in promoting patient rights

1. Communication and information

- **Active listening**: listening to patients' questions and concerns, helping them to express their needs and expectations.
- **Transmitting information**: providing clear explanations of the care provided, within the limits of its competence, and directing the patient to the nurse or doctor for more complex information.
- **Language adaptation**: Use simple language, avoid medical jargon, make sure the patient understands the information given.

2. Respecting consent

- **Ask for agreement**: Before any treatment or procedure, even a simple one, ask for the patient's agreement, briefly explaining the purpose and the procedure.
- **Observing reactions**: Pay attention to verbal and non-verbal signals indicating the patient's consent or refusal.
- **Respecting refusal**: If the patient refuses care, respect his or her decision and inform the nurse or doctor so that appropriate care can be taken.

3. Promoting autonomy

- **Encouraging participation**: Involve patients in decisions concerning their day-to-day care, promoting their autonomy wherever possible.
- **Valuing abilities**: Recognizing and supporting patients' skills, however small, to boost their self-confidence.

4. Privacy policy

- **Discretion**: Ensure confidentiality of exchanges, avoid divulging personal information to unauthorized third parties.
- **Document management** : Handle patient files and documents with care, respecting confidentiality protocols.

5. Respect for dignity

- **Equal treatment**: Offer the same care and attention to all patients, without discrimination based on age, gender, origin, religion or any other characteristic.
- **Professional behavior**: Adopt a respectful, empathetic and caring attitude in all circumstances.

Informed consent in practice

1. Definition and importance

Informed consent is the process by which a patient accepts treatment or care after having received adequate information about it. It is essential to respect the patient's autonomy and right to control his or her own body.

2. Informed consent process

- **Prior information**: Patients must be given all necessary information about the proposed care or treatment, including expected benefits, potential risks, possible alternatives and the consequences of refusal.

- ◦ **Comprehension**: Ensure that the patient has understood the information given, by checking comprehension and answering questions.
- ◦ **Free will**: Consent must be given without coercion, pressure or manipulation.
- ◦ **Legal capacity**: The patient must be legally capable of giving consent (adult, conscious, no impairment of discernment). For minors or protected adults, legal representatives are involved.

3. The caregiver's role in informed consent

- ◦ **Communication support**: Facilitating dialogue between the patient and the medical team, helping the patient to formulate questions or concerns.
- ◦ **Observation**: Tell the nurse or doctor if the patient seems not to have understood the information or shows signs of anxiety or confusion.
- ◦ **Respecting the patient's choice**: Whatever the patient's decision, the caregiver must respect it and continue care within the defined framework.

Challenges and complex situations

1. Non-communicative or vulnerable patients

- ◦ **Impaired consciousness**: For patients who are unconscious or unable to communicate, decisions are made in accordance with advance directives, previously expressed wishes or in consultation with the family.
- ◦ **Cognitive disorders**: With patients suffering from dementia or psychiatric disorders, it's important to

assess their ability to understand and consent, by adapting communication.

2. Medical emergencies

- ○ **Presumed consent**: In life-threatening emergencies, when the patient is unable to give consent, the necessary care is provided in his or her best interests, following established protocols.

3. Refusal of care

- ○ **Respect for refusal**: If a patient refuses care, even if this refusal may have serious consequences, his or her decision must be respected after ensuring that he or she is properly informed.
- ○ **Communication with the team**: Inform the nurse or doctor of the refusal so that they can assess the situation and offer appropriate support.

Training and awareness-raising

- **Knowledge of patient rights**: Caregivers must be trained in patient rights, legal and ethical aspects, so as to integrate them into their daily practice.
- **Development of communication skills**: Improve your ability to convey information, listen actively and adapt your language to the patient.
- **Ethical reflection**: Participate in ethical discussions, discussion groups or training courses to deepen your understanding of issues related to patient rights.

Concrete examples to illustrate the principles

1. Request for information about a treatment

Mrs Lefèvre is due to receive a subcutaneous injection. She expresses her fear and incomprehension about the need for this procedure.

- ○ **Caregiver's approach**: Calmly explain the purpose of the injection, the expected benefits, reassure her about the procedure, and check if she would like further information from the nurse.

2. Patient refuses bath

Mr Bernard refuses to wash in the morning, feeling tired.

- ○ **Caregiver's approach**: Respect her refusal, suggest an alternative (toilet later in the day, partial toilet), and inform the nurse of the situation.

- • Professional practices and legal responsibilities

The profession of nursing auxiliary in internal medicine is governed by rigorous professional practices and specific legal responsibilities. These frameworks define not only the technical skills required, but also the ethical, moral and legal obligations that accompany every gesture, every decision and every interaction with the patient. Understanding and integrating these principles is essential to providing quality care, protecting patients' rights, and ensuring that practice conforms to established standards. This chapter explores in depth the professional practices expected of caregivers, as well as the legal responsibilities that flow from them, emphasizing the importance of ethics, continuing education and personal reflection in the daily practice of this profession.

The foundations of professional practice

The caregiver's professional practices are guided by a set of standards and values designed to ensure the safety, well-being and dignity of patients. They are based on :

1. Technical expertise

- ○ **Mastery of gestures** : Caregivers must have the technical skills required to carry out the care tasks entrusted to them, in compliance with established protocols and procedures.

- ◦ **Updating knowledge**: Keeping abreast of scientific, technological and regulatory developments is essential to maintaining a high level of competence.

2. Professional ethics

- ◦ **Respect for the individual**: Every patient must be treated with respect, without discrimination, recognizing his or her dignity and rights.
- ◦ **Beneficence and non-maleficence**: The caregiver must act in the patient's interest, avoiding causing harm.
- ◦ **Justice**: Providing equitable care for all patients, by distributing resources fairly.

3. Communication

- ◦ **Clarity and honesty**: Communicating transparently with patients and the care team.
- ◦ **Active listening**: Listening to patients' needs, concerns and expectations.

4. Interprofessional collaboration

- ◦ **Teamwork**: Collaborate effectively with nurses, doctors and other healthcare professionals to ensure comprehensive patient care.
- ◦ **Information sharing**: Transmit relevant information in an accurate and timely manner.

The caregiver's legal responsibilities

Caregivers are subject to legal obligations that govern their professional practice. These responsibilities are designed to protect the patient, the professional and the healthcare institution.

134

1. Respect for the practice environment

- ○ **Competence limits**: Caregivers must know which procedures they are authorized to perform, and which are the exclusive responsibility of nurses or doctors.
- ○ **Delegation of tasks**: When acting under the nurse's delegation, the nurse must respect instructions and not exceed his/her duties.

2. Safety obligation

- ○ **Risk prevention**: Apply hygiene and safety measures to prevent nosocomial infections, accidents and medication errors.
- ○ **Professional vigilance**: Monitor the patient's condition and report any anomalies or significant changes.

3. Professional secrecy

- ○ **Confidentiality**: Protect the patient's personal and medical information, while respecting medical confidentiality.
- ○ **Criminal liability**: Breach of professional secrecy is punishable by law and may result in criminal penalties.

4. Duty of care

- ○ **Non-assistance to a person in danger**: Caregivers have a legal obligation to assist a person in danger, acting within the limits of their competence and alerting the appropriate emergency services.

5. Traceability and documentation

- ○ **Record-keeping**: Participate in documenting the care provided, in compliance with traceability procedures.
- ○ **Accuracy of information** : Ensure that recorded information is accurate, complete and truthful.

Ethical principles guiding practice

1. Patient autonomy

- ○ **Respect for choice**: Patients have the right to make decisions about their own health. Caregivers must respect these choices, even if they differ from their own convictions.
- ○ **Informed consent**: Ensuring that the patient is adequately informed to consent to care.

2. Charity

- ○ **Acting for the patient's well-being**: All actions must aim to improve the patient's well-being, relieve suffering and promote health.

3. Non-maleficence

- ○ **Do no harm**: Do no harm to the patient, whether by action or omission.

4. Justice

- ○ **Fairness**: Treat all patients equally, without favoritism or discrimination.

5. Loyalty

- ○ **Commitment**: Honor promises made to patients, respect agreements and maintain trust.

136

Specific legal obligations

1. **Civil liability**

   ○ **Compensation for damage**: In the event of malpractice causing damage to the patient, the orderly may be required to pay compensation for the damage suffered.

2. **Criminal liability**

   ○ **Criminal offences**: acts such as gross negligence, maltreatment or breach of medical confidentiality may render the caregiver criminally liable.

3. **Disciplinary liability**

   ○ **Professional sanctions**: Failure to comply with professional rules may result in disciplinary action by the employer or professional bodies.

Ongoing training and professional development

1. **Updating knowledge**

   ○ **Mandatory continuing education**: Participate in continuing education programs to maintain and develop your skills.
   ○ **Professional watch**: Keep abreast of legislative, scientific and technical developments.

2. **Ethical reflection**

   ○ **Discussion groups**: Participate in discussions on ethical dilemmas encountered in practice.
   ○ **Supervision**: Benefit from support to reflect on your practice and experiences.

3. Personal commitment

- **Self-evaluation**: Regularly reflect on your practice, identifying strengths and areas for improvement.
- **Developing soft skills**: Improving communication, stress management and teamwork skills.

Challenges and possible solutions

1. Institutional pressure

- **High workload**: Managing stress and fatigue to maintain optimum quality of care.
- **Lack of resources**: Demonstrate creativity and adaptability to offer quality care despite constraints.

2. Ethical conflicts

- **Moral dilemmas**: Dealing with situations where legal and ethical obligations and the patient's interests may be in conflict.
- **Institutional support**: Use available resources, such as ethics committees, for advice and support.

3. Error management

- **Acknowledging mistakes**: Admitting mistakes, understanding their causes and taking steps to correct them.
- **Transparency**: Inform the care team and, if necessary, the patient, in compliance with institutional procedures.

The caregiver's role in promoting quality of care

1. **Participation in continuous improvement**

   ○ **Reporting undesirable events**: Help identify risks and implement preventive measures.
   ○ **Suggestions for improvement**: sharing ideas for optimizing practices and processes.

2. **Interprofessional collaboration**

   ○ **Teamwork**: Foster open and respectful communication with other professionals.
   ○ **Knowledge sharing**: Contribute to the training of new team members, share best practices.

3. **Commitment to patients**

   ○ **Patient-centricity**: Putting the patient at the heart of our concerns, adapting care to his or her specific needs.
   ○ **Promoting patient rights**: Ensuring that patients' rights are respected, informing them and supporting them in their decisions.

Concrete examples illustrating professional practices and legal responsibilities

1. **Respecting professional boundaries**
   Mr. Dubois asks the orderly to administer an injectable medication in the nurse's absence.

   ○ **Appropriate response**: Explain to Mr. Dubois that the administration of injectable medications is the nurse's responsibility and that, for his safety, it is important to respect this rule. Inform the nurse of the patient's request for appropriate management.

2. **Reporting an adverse event**
The orderly notices an error in the distribution of medication: a tablet has been given to the wrong patient.

   ○ **Action to be undertaken**: Immediately inform the nurse in charge, monitor the patient's condition, and participate in reporting the incident according to internal procedures, with the aim of improving care safety.

• Compliance with safety protocols and standards
Compliance with protocols and safety standards is an essential pillar in the practice of the internal medicine orderly. These guidelines guarantee not only the safety and well-being of patients, but also that of caregivers and all hospital staff. They provide the framework that guides daily actions, ensures quality of care and prevents the risk of accidents or infections. This chapter explores in depth the importance of compliance with these protocols, the responsibilities of the caregiver in implementing them, and the impact they have on the quality of care and safety within the healthcare establishment.

The importance of compliance with safety protocols and standards

Safety protocols and standards are established for :

• **Ensuring patient safety**: Avoiding medical errors, nosocomial infections and care-related accidents.
• **Protecting caregivers**: Prevent workplace accidents and exposure to infectious or chemical agents.
• **Guaranteeing quality of care**: providing services in line with best practice, based on scientific evidence.

- **Comply with legal obligations**: Comply with national and international regulations and the recommendations of health authorities.

Compliance with these guidelines is therefore a major responsibility for caregivers, who must integrate them into their daily practice and understand what is at stake.

The fundamentals of safety protocols and standards

1. **Standardizing practices**

    Protocols help to standardize care, by defining clear procedures for each act. This reduces undesirable variations in practices, decreases the risk of errors and facilitates coordination between members of the care team.

2. **Risk prevention**

    Safety standards are designed to identify and control potential risks to patients and caregivers. They include measures to prevent infection, manage waste, handle equipment safely, and respond to emergencies.

3. **Continuous improvement**

    Protocols are regularly updated to incorporate scientific advances, new technologies and feedback. The nursing auxiliary must therefore keep abreast of developments and play an active role in improving practices.

The caregiver's role in respecting protocols

1. **Rigorous application of procedures**

    The nursing auxiliary is responsible for carrying out care according to established protocols. This involves :

    - **Know the protocols**: Read documents carefully, take part in training sessions, ask questions when in doubt.

- Follow prescribed steps: Respect the order of actions, use recommended techniques, check control points.
- Use the right equipment: select the right equipment, check that it is working properly, report any malfunctions.

2. **Monitoring and preventing incidents**

Caregivers must be alert to signs of risk or malfunction:

- Patient observation: Look for signs of infection, pain, adverse reactions.
- Environmental control: Ensure that areas are clean, clear and safe.
- Incident reporting : Immediately report any undesirable event, however minor, to enable rapid intervention.

3. **Collaboration with the care team**

Compliance with protocols is a collective responsibility:

- Effective communication: passing on relevant information, sharing observations, coordinating actions.
- Mutual support: helping colleagues to comply with procedures, exchanging best practices.
- Participation in meetings: Contribute to discussions on protocols, suggest improvements based on field experience.

Application of protocols in daily practice

1. **Hand hygiene**

- Appropriate technique: Wash with soap and water or hydroalcoholic rub as indicated.

- **Key times**: Before and after each contact with the patient, before an aseptic procedure, after a risk of exposure to biological fluids.
- **Awareness**: Encourage patients and visitors to practice good hand hygiene.

2. Use of personal protective equipment (PPE)

- **Wearing gloves, masks and gowns**: According to standard precautions and additional precautions.
- **Removal and disposal**: Remove PPE safely to avoid contamination, dispose of in appropriate channels.
- **Maintenance of reusable equipment**: Clean and disinfect in accordance with protocols.

3. Waste and linen management

- **Selective sorting**: Separate infectious, sharp and recyclable waste according to defined categories.
- **Safe handling**: Use suitable containers, avoid overloading, close bags properly.
- **Transport and storage**: Follow designated routes to avoid cross-contamination.

4. Technical care safety

- **Material preparation**: Check sterility, expiration date, packaging integrity.
- **Asepsis**: Respect aseptic techniques during invasive care (catheter insertion, dressings).
- **Medication administration**: Respect the 5Bs (Right patient, Right drug, Right dose, Right route, Right time), even if the caregiver does not administer them directly.

5. Falls and accident prevention

- **Risk assessment**: Identify patients at risk of falling, adapt environment (bed rails, lighting).
- **Mobility assistance**: Use safe handling techniques and technical aids (walkers, wheelchairs).
- **Training**: Participate in training courses on accident prevention and load handling.

The different safety domains

1. Patient safety

- **Correct identification**: Check the patient's identity before any treatment or examination.
- **Error prevention**: Double-checking prescriptions, compliance with double-checking protocols.
- **Clinical monitoring**: Observe vital signs, reactions to treatment, report any abnormalities.

2. Caregiver safety

- **Infection prevention**: Observe standard precautions, protect yourself during high-risk treatments.
- **Physical safety**: using protective equipment, adopting ergonomic postures to avoid musculoskeletal disorders.
- **Stress management**: Recognize signs of fatigue, overload, take necessary breaks.

3. **Environmental safety**

- ○ **Maintenance of premises**: Participate in the cleanliness of the premises, report any damage or anomalies.
- ○ **Equipment management**: Ensure that equipment is in good condition, report breakdowns and avoid inappropriate use.
- ○ **Emergency preparedness**: evacuation plans, fire and disaster procedures.

The importance of ongoing training and awareness-raising

1. **Updating knowledge**

- ○ **Participate in training courses**: mandatory or complementary, on protocols, safety standards, new practices.
- ○ **Stay informed**: Read internal communications, postings, protocol updates.

2. **Skills development**

- ○ **Practical workshops**: training in technical gestures and the use of new equipment.
- ○ **Professional exchanges**: discussing with colleagues, sharing experiences, difficulties and solutions found.

3. **Raising awareness of the issues**

- ○ **Understand the impact**: Recognize the importance of protocol compliance on safety, quality of care and patient satisfaction.

- ○ **Personal commitment**: Adopt a proactive attitude, be a role model for colleagues, encourage compliance with standards.

Challenges encountered and strategies for overcoming them

1. High workload

- ○ **Efficient organization**: Plan tasks, prioritize actions, avoid rushing, which can lead to mistakes.
- ○ **Asking for help**: Don't hesitate to ask your colleagues or manager if you're overloaded.

2. Lack of resources

- ○ **Rational management**: Use resources appropriately, avoid waste.
- ○ **Reporting**: Inform hierarchy of material requirements and stock shortages.

3. Resistance to change

- ○ **Training**: Understanding the reasons behind the new standards and the expected benefits.
- ○ **Communication**: express concerns, suggest improvements, participate in working groups.

The impact of protocol compliance on quality of care

- **Reduced nosocomial infections**: fewer pathogens transmitted, improved patient health.
- **Fewer medical errors**: less risk of confusion, incorrect administration and accidents.
- **Improved patient satisfaction**: Sense of security, confidence in the care team.
- **Enhancing the facility's reputation**: positive image, attractiveness to patients and professionals.

Chapter 7

Challenges in the Internal Medicine Department

- Workload and time management

Workload and time management are major issues for the internal medicine orderly. In a hospital environment where patients' needs are complex and varied, the orderly is often faced with a multitude of tasks to accomplish within tight deadlines. The ability to manage time effectively, prioritize actions and maintain a balance between quality of care and organizational requirements is essential to ensure optimal service to patients while preserving one's own professional well-being. This chapter explores workload challenges, time management strategies and the importance of a balanced approach to ensuring sustainable and satisfying professional practice.

Workload challenges in Internal Medicine

1. Complex care

- **Multiplicity of tasks**: The caregiver must carry out a variety of direct care tasks (toileting, assistance with feeding, mobilization) and indirect care tasks (preparation of equipment, transmission of information).
- **Patients with special needs**: Internal Medicine welcomes patients with various pathologies, often chronic or serious, requiring special attention.

2. Time pressure

- **Tight deadlines**: Care must be carried out within precise time slots, respecting mealtimes, medical examinations and visiting hours.
- **Unforeseen emergencies**: Critical situations can arise at any time, upsetting the established schedule.

3. **Limited workforce**

   ○ **Understaffing**: The number of caregivers may be insufficient for the number of patients, increasing individual workloads.
   ○ **Absences and replacements**: Leave, sick leave or training can create gaps in the team.

4. **Administrative requirements**

   ○ **Documentation**: Record-keeping, care traceability and incident reporting are time-consuming and demanding.
   ○ **Meetings and training**: Taking part in team meetings and mandatory training courses adds to our obligations.

The consequences of an excessive workload

1. **Compromised quality of care**

   ○ **Risk of errors**: Fatigue and haste can lead to oversights or errors in care.
   ○ **Less attention to patients**: Lack of time reduces availability for listening and supporting patients.

2. **Stress and burnout**

   ○ **Burn-out**: Accumulated stress can lead to physical and emotional exhaustion, affecting the caregiver's health.
   ○ **Job dissatisfaction**: The feeling of not being able to do one's job properly can reduce motivation and commitment.

3. **Strained interpersonal relations**

   ○ **Team conflicts**: Pressure can generate tension between colleagues, affecting collaboration.

- ○ **Impaired communication**: Lack of time can reduce the quality of exchanges with patients and the care team.

Time management strategies for caregivers

1. Planning and organization

- ○ **Establish a daily schedule**: Prioritize tasks according to urgency and importance, taking into account patient needs and time constraints.
- ○ **Use tools**: To-do lists, tracking charts and mobile apps can help you organize your work.

2. Prioritizing tasks

- ○ **Identify priorities**: Focus first on care essential to patient safety and comfort.
- ○ **Delegate where possible**: Collaborate with colleagues to share tasks, ask for help when overloaded.

3. Interrupt management

- ○ **Limit distractions**: Avoid non-essential interruptions, group similar tasks together to save time.
- ○ **Managing emergencies**: adapting to the unexpected while maintaining a global vision of priorities.

4. Optimizing travel

- ○ **Group care by sector**: Avoid unnecessary round trips by planning care in the same area.
- ○ **Material preparation**: Anticipate material requirements to avoid wasting time.

5. **Effective communication**

- ○ **Clear communication**: Provide and receive precise information during shift changes to avoid oversights.
- ○ **Short, focused meetings**: Optimize meeting time by concentrating on the essential points.

Practices to improve time management

1. **Self-evaluation**

- ○ **Analyze your schedule**: Identify the tasks that take up the most time, the sources of delay or stress.
- ○ **Identify areas for improvement**: reflect on ways to improve efficiency.

2. **Training and skills development**

- ○ **Participate in training courses**: Learn time management, communication and problem-solving techniques.
- ○ **Sharing best practices**: exchanging effective strategies and time management tips with colleagues.

3. **Stress management**

- ○ **Relaxation techniques**: use breathing and mindfulness exercises to stay calm and focused.
- ○ **Work-life balance**: Take breaks, respect rest periods, engage in relaxing activities outside work.

4. **Collaboration and team spirit**

- ○ **Solidarity between colleagues**: helping each other out, sharing the load, creating a positive dynamic within the team.

- ○ **Open communication**: expressing needs and difficulties, proposing collective solutions.

The importance of institutional support

1. **The role of management and healthcare executives**

- ○ **Workload assessment**: Regularly analyze workloads to adapt staffing levels.
- ○ **Putting resources in place**: providing tools, training and support for teams.

2. **Process improvement**

- ○ **Simplification of procedures**: Reduce redundant administrative tasks, optimize circuits.
- ○ **Introduction of technologies**: Use computer systems to facilitate documentation and communication.

3. **Promoting well-being at work**

- ○ **Burn-out prevention programs**: offering psychological support services and stress management workshops.
- ○ **Work recognition**: Valuing caregivers' efforts, celebrating successes, fostering a positive work climate.

Case study: Application of time management strategies

Mrs. Dupont, a nurse's aide in Internal Medicine, feels overwhelmed by her daily tasks. She decides to apply strategies to improve her time management.

- • **Planning**: She starts her day by drawing up a list of priority tasks, taking into account the specific needs of patients.

- **Optimizing travel**: She groups treatments by room, preparing the necessary equipment in advance.
- **Collaboration**: She coordinates with her colleagues to share heavy tasks, such as mobilizing dependent patients.
- **Interruption management**: She informs the team that she will be available for non-urgent matters after completing critical care.
- **Self-evaluation**: At the end of the day, she reflects on the positive points and possible improvements for the following day.

After a few weeks, Ms Dupont noticed a reduction in stress, greater efficiency in her tasks and greater job satisfaction.

- Adapting to technological and medical developments

The world of healthcare is constantly changing, marked by technological and medical advances that are profoundly transforming care practices. For the internal medicine orderly, this constant evolution represents both a challenge and an opportunity. It is essential to adapt in order to remain relevant, efficient and offer quality care to patients. This chapter explores the challenges of this adaptation, the skills needed to integrate new technologies, and strategies for successfully navigating this changing landscape.

The impact of technological developments on healthcare practice

Medical technologies have revolutionized the way care is delivered. From innovative medical devices to sophisticated information systems, these tools have the potential to improve the quality of care, increase efficiency and facilitate communication between healthcare professionals.

1. Advanced medical devices

- **Vital signs monitors**: Modern devices enable continuous, precise monitoring of vital parameters, quickly alerting the care team to any abnormality.
- **Intelligent infusion pumps**: They ensure precise drug delivery, reducing the risk of errors and improving patient safety.
- **Assistive mobility technologies**: automated medical beds, electric patient lifts and exoskeletons facilitate patient mobilization while preserving the physical health of caregivers.

2. Information and communication systems

- **Computerized patient files (DPI)**: These centralize medical information, facilitating access to relevant data and improving care coordination.
- **Mobile and tablet applications**: These tools enable real-time recording of the care provided, rapid consultation of protocols and fluid communication between team members.
- **Telecare and telemedicine**: These offer new possibilities for remote monitoring, specialist consultation and therapeutic education.

3. Artificial intelligence and automation

- **Predictive algorithms**: These help identify at-risk patients, enabling early intervention.
- **Assistive robots**: In certain contexts, they can support caregivers in repetitive or physically demanding tasks.

The challenges of adapting to new technologies

1. Training and skills

- ○ **Acquiring new skills**: Integrating complex technologies requires appropriate training to master their use and understand their clinical implications.
- ○ **Evolving roles**: The caregiver's tasks may change, necessitating a redefinition of responsibilities and skills.

2. Resistance to change

- ○ **Fear of the unknown**: The introduction of new technologies can give rise to apprehension, linked to the fear of not mastering the tools or seeing one's role diminished.
- ○ **Established habits**: Entrenched practices can make it difficult to adopt new methods.

3. Impact on the caregiver-patient relationship

- ○ **Risk of dehumanization**: The interposition of technology can affect the quality of human interaction, an essential element of care.
- ○ **Patient adaptation**: Some patients may be reluctant or have difficulty interacting with technologies, requiring specific support.

Strategies for successful adaptation

1. Continuing education and professional development

- ○ **Training programs**: Actively participate in training programs offered by the company, whether technical or focused on interpersonal skills in a technological context.

- ○ **Self-training**: Use online resources, tutorials and manuals to deepen your knowledge.

2. Proactive, open approach

- ○ **Curiosity and enthusiasm**: Adopt a positive attitude to innovation, seeing technologies as opportunities for improvement.
- ○ **Sharing experiences**: exchanging views with colleagues on challenges encountered, solutions found and best practices.

3. Interprofessional collaboration

- ○ **Teamwork**: Work closely with nurses, doctors and technicians to ensure smooth integration of technologies.
- ○ **Involvement in projects**: Participate in committees and working groups on the implementation of new technologies, bringing your own perspective.

4. Patient focus

- ○ **Humanizing care**: Ensuring that technology does not replace listening, empathy and human contact.
- ○ **Patient support**: Helping patients to understand and accept the technologies used in their care, answering their questions and allaying their concerns.

Key skills for the modern caregiver

1. Technical skills

- ○ **Mastering digital tools**: knowing how to use software, applications and connected medical devices.

- Understanding **technological protocols**: Knowing the specific procedures involved in using new technologies, security protocols and data protection.

2. Interpersonal skills

- **Appropriate communication**: Clearly explain the use of technology to patients, in terms they can understand.
- **Technological empathy**: understanding patients' reluctance or difficulties with technology, adapting your support.

3. Problem-solving skills

- **Adaptability**: Be able to react quickly to malfunctions, find solutions or request appropriate help.
- **Critical thinking**: Evaluate the effectiveness of technologies, suggest improvements, point out problems.

Ethical and regulatory issues

1. Personal data protection

- **Confidentiality**: Ensuring the security of digitized medical information, respecting confidentiality protocols.
- **Legal compliance**: Comply with data protection laws, such as the General Data Protection Regulation (GDPR).

2. **Fair access**

   ○ **Combating inequalities**: Ensuring that all patients benefit from technological advances, regardless of their social, economic or cultural situation.
   ○ **Cultural adaptation**: taking into account cultural specificities in the use of technologies, respecting patients' beliefs and preferences.

3. **Maintaining professional autonomy**

   ○ **Role of clinical judgment**: Don't rely solely on technology, but use your expertise to interpret data and make informed decisions.
   ○ **Ethical training**: Participate in training courses on the ethical challenges of technologies, to integrate these considerations into daily practice.

The positive impact of technology on care

1. **Improved quality of care**

   ○ **Accuracy and reliability**: technologies reduce errors and enable more precise patient follow-up.
   ○ **Personalized care**: the data collected enables care to be tailored to the specific needs of each patient.

2. **Operational efficiency**

   ○ **Time savings**: automating certain tasks frees up time for direct care.
   ○ **Fluid communication**: Information systems facilitate the sharing of information and coordination between professionals.

3. Professional development

- ○ **Skills development**: Learning new technologies enriches career paths and opens up new career prospects.
- ○ **Professional recognition**: mastery of technology can enhance the role of the caregiver within the care team.

Case study: Integrating a new computerized patient record system

When a hospital decides to implement a new computerized patient record system, the orderly is faced with several challenges:

- **Initial training**: He takes part in organized training sessions, takes notes, and doesn't hesitate to ask questions to clarify complex points.
- **Progressive practice**: using the system under the supervision of an experienced colleague, practicing data entry and consulting the necessary information.
- **Adapting routines**: adjusting the way they work, integrating the use of the system into their daily tasks, optimizing time by combining actions.
- **Colleague support**: Sharing tips and tricks, helping colleagues in difficulty, contributing to a climate of mutual support.
- **Constructive feedback**: identifies problems and suggests improvements to make the system easier to use.

Thanks to this proactive approach, the caregiver not only adapts effectively to the new system, but also contributes to its success and to improved patient care.

- Occupational risk prevention

Occupational risk prevention is an essential part of the nursing auxiliary's job in internal medicine. Working in direct contact with patients and confronted with a variety of potentially dangerous situations, orderlies must be aware of the risks to which they are exposed in order to protect their health, ensure their safety and maintain optimum quality of care. This chapter explores the different types of occupational hazards, strategies for preventing them, and the importance of a safety culture within the care team.

Types of occupational hazards in internal medicine

1. **Biological risks**

   Nurses are exposed to a variety of infectious agents when caring for patients:

   - **Exposure to pathogens**: Bacteria, viruses and fungi can be transmitted by direct or indirect contact.
   - **Accidents involving exposure to blood (AES)**: Punctures, cuts or splashes of biological fluids carry a risk of transmitting diseases such as HIV, hepatitis B or C.

2. **Chemical hazards**

   - **Handling chemicals**: Disinfectants, detergents, cytotoxic drugs can cause irritation, allergies or poisoning.
   - **Aerosol exposure**: Inhalation of particles when preparing or administering certain treatments.

3. **Physical hazards**

   - **Musculoskeletal disorders (MSD)**: Repetitive movements, awkward postures, handling heavy

loads (patient transfers) lead to back, shoulder and joint pain and injury.
- **Ionizing radiation** : Exposure during certain radiological examinations.

4. Psychosocial risks

- **Stress and burnout**: heavy workloads, staggered working hours, confrontation with suffering and death can lead to burn-out.
- **Violence and aggression**: Patients or visitors may behave aggressively, either verbally or physically.

5. Organizational risks

- **Lack of staff**: Increases individual workload, stress, risk of errors.
- **Lack of training**: Insufficient or inadequate training can lead to misapplication of safety protocols.

Risk prevention strategies

1. Training and awareness-raising

- **Ongoing training programs**: Regular participation in training courses on hygiene, handling, stress management and emergency procedures.
- **Updating knowledge**: Keep abreast of new recommendations, protocols and best practices.

2. Rigorous application of hygiene protocols

- **Hand hygiene**: Practice handwashing or disinfection by hydro-alcoholic friction according to the five WHO indications.

○ **Use of personal protective equipment (PPE)**: Wear gloves, masks, goggles, smocks when necessary.

3. Prevention of blood exposure accidents

○ **Use safe equipment**: Use devices with built-in safety devices to prevent accidental pricks.
○ **Infectious risk waste management**: Properly dispose of needles and sharps in suitable containers.

4. Ergonomics and safe handling

○ **Patient mobilization techniques**: Apply ergonomic transfer methods, use technical aids such as patient lifts or sliding sheets.
○ **Work environment layout**: Organize space to reduce unnecessary physical effort, adjust the height of beds and carts.

5. Psychosocial risk management

○ **Developing communication skills**: learning to defuse conflict situations, adopting an empathetic attitude.
○ **Psychological support**: Access support services, take part in discussion groups, share experiences with colleagues.
○ **Work-life balance**: Take regular breaks, enjoy relaxing activities outside work, look after your health.

6. Compliance with safety procedures

○ **Hazard warning**: Inform the team of any identified hazards, such as slippery floors or faulty equipment.

- ○ **Participation in safety drills**: taking part in fire simulations and emergency plan training.

The importance of a safety culture

1. Collective responsibility

- ○ **Team commitment**: Risk prevention is everyone's business. Each team member must be vigilant and support the others in applying safety measures.
- ○ **Open communication**: Foster an environment where everyone can report incidents or near-misses without fear of blame.

2. Institutional support

- ○ **Prevention policies**: The facility must put in place clear policies, accessible protocols and sufficient resources for risk prevention.
- ○ **Investment in equipment**: Provide high-quality personal protective equipment and technical aids for handling.

3. Assessment and continuous improvement

- ○ **Incident analysis**: Study accidents to understand the causes and implement corrective actions.
- ○ **Updating practices**: Adapting protocols in line with feedback, technological advances and official recommendations.

The benefits of occupational risk prevention

- **Employee health and well-being**: Better prevention reduces work-related accidents and illnesses, and improves quality of life at work.
- **Quality of care**: Healthy, safe caregivers are better able to provide quality care to patients.

- **Reduced costs**: Fewer accidents mean less absenteeism, lower care costs for injured carers, and lower compensation costs.
- **Positive work climate**: A culture of safety strengthens trust between team members, promotes collaboration and job satisfaction.

Case studies

1. Preventing needlestick accidents

While taking a blood sample, an orderly is injured by a used needle. To prevent this risk :

- **Use safety-engineered needles**.
- **Never recap a used needle**.
- **Dispose of the needle immediately in a suitable container**.
- **In the event of an accident**, apply HSE protocols: clean the wound, report the incident, carry out the necessary examinations.

2. Managing stress in an aggressive patient

A confused patient becomes agitated and threatening.

- **Maintain a safe distance**.
- **Speak calmly**, using short, reassuring sentences.
- **Call for back-up** if necessary.
- **After the incident**, debrief the team, identify triggers and plan strategies to avoid similar situations in the future.

- Work-life balance

The profession of internal medicine orderly is demanding, both physically and psychologically. Irregular working hours, night shifts, the emotional burden of caring for patients who are often seriously ill, as well as administrative demands, can make it difficult to reconcile professional and personal life. Yet striking this balance is essential not only for the caregiver's well-being, but also for the quality of patient care. This chapter explores the challenges inherent in this profession and suggests strategies for maintaining a healthy work-life balance.

The challenges of work-life balance in Internal Medicine

The job of a nurse's aide in internal medicine is characterized by intense working days, when patients' needs are multiple and complex. Staggered working hours, often including nights, weekends and public holidays, disrupt biological rhythms and can affect social and family life. What's more, the emotional burden of caring for patients with chronic illnesses or at the end of life can lead to significant psychological fatigue.

Administrative requirements, such as record-keeping and attendance at meetings, add a further burden. Staff shortages in some departments can also increase individual workloads, making it even more difficult to switch off at the end of the day.

The consequences of work-life imbalance

Prolonged imbalance can have negative repercussions on the caregiver's physical and mental health. Possible consequences include:

- **Chronic fatigue**: lack of rest and disruption of sleep cycles can lead to persistent fatigue, affecting alertness and performance at work.

- **Stress and burn-out**: The accumulation of stress without adequate recovery periods can lead to burn-out, characterized by emotional fatigue, depersonalization and a sense of diminished personal fulfillment.

- **Health problems**: Constant stress can increase the risk of cardiovascular, musculoskeletal and immune disorders.

- **Impact on personal life**: Family and social relationships can suffer, with less time spent with loved ones, which can lead to feelings of isolation or guilt.

- **Decreased quality of care**: An exhausted caregiver may find it difficult to maintain the same quality of attention and compassion towards patients, which can affect the caregiver-patient relationship.

Strategies for achieving a healthy balance

1. **Time and priority management**

    ○ **Proactive planning**: Organize your schedule to take into account professional and personal obligations. Use a diary to note work schedules, personal appointments and rest periods.

    ○ **Setting priorities**: Identify what is essential at work and at home, and devote time to these activities. Learn to say no to requests that are not priorities.

2. **Taking care of your physical health**

    ○ **Quality sleep**: Create an environment conducive to sleep, especially after night shifts. As far as possible, maintain a regular sleep pattern.

    ○ **Balanced diet**: Eat healthily to maintain energy and health. Prepare meals in advance to avoid junk food when you're tired or short of time.

    ○ **Regular physical activity**: Incorporate exercise into your routine, even in short sessions, to reduce stress and improve overall well-being.

3. Stress management and mental well-being

- ○ **Relaxation techniques**: Practice meditation, yoga, deep breathing or other techniques to reduce daily stress.

- ○ **Moments of disconnection**: Take time out from the phone and work e-mails to refocus on yourself or spend quality time with loved ones.

- ○ **Pleasurable activities**: Devoting time to hobbies or activities that bring pleasure and personal satisfaction.

4. Maintaining social and family relationships

- ○ **Open communication**: Sharing the challenges and constraints of the job with family and friends to foster mutual understanding.

- ○ **Quality rather than quantity**: Make the most of time spent with family and friends, by being present and attentive.

- ○ **Mutual support**: Participate in support groups or activities with colleagues to share experiences and advice.

5. Setting professional boundaries

- ○ **Work-life separation**: Avoid taking work home with you. If possible, complete administrative tasks before leaving the office.

- ○ **Solicitation management**: Don't feel obliged to answer business calls or messages outside working hours, except in emergencies.

6. Use available resources

- **Workplace wellness programs**: Take advantage of services offered by the facility, such as stress management workshops, sports sessions or psychological consultations.

- **Ongoing training**: Take part in training courses on time management, personal development or communication to improve your skills and job satisfaction.

7. Involving the team and management

- **Communication with superiors**: Express your needs and difficulties to managers, and seek appropriate solutions, such as flexible working hours or additional support.

- **Collaboration between colleagues**: helping each other to share the workload fairly, cover absences, and create a positive work climate.

The importance of self-compassion

It's essential to be kind to yourself. Acknowledging your limits, accepting that you can't control everything, and avoiding blaming yourself when things go wrong all help to preserve your mental health. Taking a step back from stressful situations and remembering the reasons why you chose this profession can restore meaning and motivation.

The role of the healthcare facility

Hospitals and internal medicine departments also have a role to play in promoting work-life balance:

- **Scheduling**: Offer flexible schedules, facilitate the exchange of shifts between colleagues, limit unscheduled overtime.

- **Recognition of work**: Valuing the efforts of care assistants, offering opportunities for professional development, fostering a respectful and caring work environment.

- **Psychological support**: Providing resources to help caregivers deal with the stress and emotions associated with their work.

Chapter 8

Innovative technologies in internal medicine

- The impact of telemedicine on the role of the caregiver

Telemedicine, defined as the use of information and communication technologies to provide remote medical care, has significantly transformed the healthcare landscape in recent years. It offers opportunities to improve access to care, reduce costs and optimize available resources. In this context, the role of the caregiver is evolving to adapt to these new practices. This chapter explores how telemedicine influences the role of the caregiver, the skills required, the challenges to be met, and the opportunities it offers for improving the quality of care.

Telemedicine is changing the medical landscape

Telemedicine encompasses such diverse practices as teleconsultation, tele-expertise, telemonitoring and teleassistance. It enables patients to consult healthcare professionals without having to travel, which is particularly beneficial for people living in rural areas or with mobility difficulties. This technological evolution is changing not only the relationship between patient and doctor, but also the role of other healthcare professionals, including care assistants.

New responsibilities for caregivers

1. **Assistance during teleconsultations**

   Caregivers may be called upon to assist patients during teleconsultations, helping them to use the necessary equipment such as tablets, computers or connected medical devices. In this way, they facilitate communication between patient and doctor, ensuring that the remote consultation runs smoothly.

2. **Health data collection and transmission**

   Telemedicine often relies on the transmission of medical data in real or delayed time. The caregiver plays a key role in collecting this data, taking measurements such as blood pressure, blood sugar and oxygen saturation, and ensuring secure transmission to the relevant professionals.

172

3. Patient education and support

With the introduction of new technologies, some patients may feel unsettled. The caregiver helps them learn how to use these tools, reassures them and encourages them to take an active part in their own care. In this way, they help to reduce the digital divide and promote patient autonomy.

4. Care coordination

Telemedicine often involves increased interdisciplinary collaboration. The caregiver participates in care coordination by communicating effectively with nurses, doctors and other professionals, sharing relevant information and ensuring continuity of care.

Adapting caregiver skills

1. Mastering technological tools

Caregivers need to develop digital skills to use telemedicine devices. This includes familiarization with health data management software, teleconsultation platforms and connected medical devices.

2. Data security and confidentiality

With the handling of sensitive data, caregivers must be aware of the issues involved in protecting personal health information. They must comply with IT security protocols and current regulations, such as the General Data Protection Regulation (RGPD).

3. Remote communication

Interaction via technological means requires an adaptation of communication skills. Caregivers must learn to interpret limited non-verbal signals, express themselves clearly and build a bond of trust with the patient despite the distance.

The benefits of telemedicine for caregivers

1. **Improved quality of care**
   Telemedicine enables more regular and personalized follow-up of patients, which can improve early detection of complications and management of chronic diseases. The nursing auxiliary makes an active contribution to this improvement, providing an effective link between the patient and the medical team.

2. **Professional development**
   Adapting to telemedicine offers caregivers the opportunity to acquire new skills, which can be professionally rewarding. It also opens up prospects for career development and specialization.

3. **Flexibility and efficiency**
   Telemedicine technologies can optimize caregivers' time, reducing unnecessary travel and enabling better planning of interventions. This can contribute to better workload management and work-life balance.

The challenges and limits of telemedicine for caregivers

1. **Training and access to technology**
   Not all healthcare assistants have the required digital skills or access to the right training. It is essential that healthcare establishments invest in ongoing training to support this transition.

2. **The caregiver-patient relationship**
   Mediation by technology can sometimes alter the quality of the human relationship. The caregiver must maintain a personalized, empathetic approach, compensating for the limitations of remote interactions.

3. **Increased workload**
   The integration of new telemedicine-related tasks can increase the caregiver's workload. It is important that these

additional responsibilities are recognized and that the necessary resources are made available.

The future of the caregiver's role with telemedicine

Telemedicine is set to develop further, particularly with the rapid advances in digital technologies and the changing needs of the population. The nursing auxiliary is strategically placed to facilitate this transition, acting as the essential link between patients and the healthcare system.

1. **Participation in telemonitoring**
    The caregiver can play a key role in telemonitoring programs, helping patients to use home monitoring devices, interpreting basic data and alerting healthcare professionals when necessary.

2. **Health promotion and prevention**
    Thanks to technology, caregivers can contribute to broader prevention and health education initiatives, by taking part in online campaigns, webinars or using dedicated applications.

3. **Enhanced inter-professional collaboration**
    Telemedicine encourages networking between different healthcare professionals. Caregivers can collaborate with a wider team, benefit from exchanges of best practices and participate in innovative projects.

* Using digital tools to monitor patients

The rapid evolution of digital technologies has profoundly transformed the healthcare field, opening up new possibilities for improving patient monitoring. In internal medicine, where patients often present complex pathologies requiring constant attention, the use of digital tools has become a major asset. As a key player in the day-to-day monitoring of patients, the nursing auxiliary's role is enriched and optimized by these technologies. This chapter explores the impact of digital tools on patient monitoring, the benefits they bring, the skills required for their use, and the challenges to be met for their successful integration into nursing practice.

The rise of digital health tools

Digital tools encompass a wide range of devices and software designed to collect, analyze and share healthcare data. They include:

- **Computerized patient files (DPI)**: These centralize medical information, facilitating data access and care coordination.
- **Remote monitoring devices**: sensors, vital sign monitors, portable devices that continuously measure parameters such as heart rate, blood pressure and oxygen saturation.
- **Mobile health applications (mHealth)**: Software on smartphones or tablets that enable symptom monitoring, medication management and communication with the healthcare team.
- **Remote monitoring platforms**: Systems that collect and transmit patient data to healthcare professionals for remote monitoring.

The benefits of digital tools for patient monitoring

1. **Improved quality of care**
   Digital tools enable continuous, accurate patient monitoring, promoting early detection of abnormalities. Data collected in real time can be used to quickly adjust treatments, avoid complications and improve clinical outcomes.

2. **Optimization of time and resources**
   By automating data collection, caregivers can devote more time to direct care and patient support. Reduced

176

administrative tasks and easy access to information speed up decision-making processes.

3. **Enhanced care coordination**
Digital platforms facilitate communication between different healthcare professionals. Information is shared instantaneously, promoting a consistent, multidisciplinary approach to the care plan.

4. **Greater patient involvement**
Interactive applications and devices encourage patients to actively participate in their own monitoring. They can track the evolution of their health parameters, understand the impact of their lifestyle on their condition, and collaborate more closely with the healthcare team.

The caregiver's role in using digital tools

1. **Data collection and recording**
The orderly uses digital devices to measure vital signs and other relevant parameters. He/she ensures the accuracy of the measurements, following the protocols for using the devices, and records the data in the computerized system.

2. **Monitoring and interpreting information**
Thanks to digital tools, the caregiver can continuously monitor trends in the patient's health parameters. He or she is attentive to alerts generated by the systems and identifies significant variations requiring intervention.

3. **Communication with the nursing team**
If any anomalies are detected, the caregiver quickly informs the nurses and doctors. Digital tools facilitate the sharing of information, enabling a rapid and appropriate response.

4. **Patient education and support**
The caregiver helps patients understand how to use digital devices, guides them in their handling and encourages

them to take an active part in monitoring them. They answer patients' questions and reassure them about how the technology works.

5. **Equipment maintenance**

Ensures that the equipment is working properly, cleans it, recharges it if necessary, and reports any malfunctions to the technical department.

The skills required to use digital tools

1. **Technological proficiency**

Caregivers must be comfortable using digital devices, understand their basic operation, and know how to navigate health data management software.

2. **Ongoing training**

It's important to keep up to date with new technologies, to attend training sessions organized by the company, and to keep abreast of system updates.

3. **Precision and rigor**

The reliability of data depends on the precision of measurements and the accuracy of their recording. Caregivers must be attentive to detail, scrupulously follow protocols, and check the information entered.

4. **Communication skills**

Explaining device use to patients, reassuring them about technological concerns, and communicating effectively with the healthcare team are essential skills.

5. **Respecting confidentiality**

Handling sensitive healthcare data requires knowledge of data protection regulations (such as the RGPD) and constant vigilance to ensure the confidentiality of information.

The challenges of integrating digital tools

1. **Training and adaptation**
   Adopting new technologies can be confusing. Time and resources need to be set aside to train staff, adjust work routines and adapt to change.

2. **Equipment reliability and maintenance**
   Equipment can be subject to breakdowns or malfunctions. It is important to have effective technical support and procedures for dealing with problems quickly.

3. **Data security**
   Protection against cyber-attacks and data leaks is a major challenge. Security protocols must be put in place, and staff must be made aware of best practices.

4. **Patient acceptance**
   Some patients may be reluctant to use technology, due to a lack of confidence or understanding. Support and education are essential to encourage their acceptance.

5. **Workload**
   The integration of digital tools can initially increase workload, due to the time needed to learn and adapt. Proper planning and institutional support can mitigate this effect.

Future prospects

Technological change is rapid, and new innovations continue to emerge:

- **Artificial intelligence (AI)**: AI can help analyze patient data, predict risks and propose targeted interventions. The

179

caregiver could collaborate with these systems to refine monitoring.

- **Virtual and augmented reality**: These technologies can be used for staff training, patient rehabilitation, or to make treatment easier to understand.

- **Internet of Medical Things (IoMT)**: The integration of connected devices could offer an even more comprehensive view of patients' health status, by collecting data from a variety of devices.

- Training in new medical technologies

The rapid evolution of medical technologies has profoundly transformed the healthcare landscape. New innovations appear regularly, modifying practices, protocols and interactions between healthcare professionals and patients. For the internal medicine orderly, training in new medical technologies is essential to maintain a high level of competence, ensure quality of care and meet the expectations of an ever-changing healthcare system. This chapter explores the importance of training in new medical technologies, key areas of innovation, associated challenges and strategies for successful integration into daily practice.

The importance of training in new medical technologies

1. **Adapting to changes in the profession**

   New technologies are changing the caregiver's tasks and responsibilities. Training enables you to :

   - **Update your skills**: Incorporate new practices to stay relevant and effective.
   - **Anticipating change**: Be proactive in the face of change, rather than undergoing it.

- Enhance your role: Demonstrate your ability to evolve, thereby strengthening your position within the healthcare team.

2. Improved quality of care

Mastering innovative technologies contributes to :

- Optimize care: Use more precise and efficient tools to monitor patients.
- Enhance safety: Reduce errors with intelligent devices and warning systems.
- Personalizing support: Adapting care based on data collected by new technologies.

3. Patient satisfaction

Patients are becoming increasingly informed and aware of the technologies used in their care. Appropriate training enables caregivers to :

- Answer patients' questions: Explain how the devices work, reassure them about their use.
- Improving the patient experience: offering modern care adapted to today's expectations.

Key areas for new medical technologies

1. Connected medical devices

- Portable vital signs monitors: enable continuous, less invasive monitoring.
- Intelligent infusion pumps: Offer precise control of drug administration.
- Motion sensors: Help prevent falls by detecting unusual movements.

2. Health information systems

- ○ **Computerized patient records (CPR)**: centralize medical information and facilitate access to data.
- ○ **Mobile applications**: Help with care planning and communication between professionals.
- ○ **Care coordination platforms**: Promote teamwork and continuity of care.

3. Virtual and augmented reality technologies

- ○ **Immersive training**: Simulations for learning technical gestures in complete safety.
- ○ **Patient support**: Use for pain management and rehabilitation.

4. Artificial intelligence and big data

- ○ **Predictive analysis**: Anticipates risks, helps decision-making.
- ○ **Virtual assistants**: support professionals in administrative tasks or sorting information.

Challenges associated with training in new technologies

1. Technological barriers

- ○ **Lack of familiarity**: Some caregivers may not be comfortable with digital technologies.
- ○ **Complexity of tools**: Devices can be sophisticated, requiring in-depth training.

2. Limited resources

- **Time available**: Workload can make it difficult to attend training courses.
- **Institutional support**: establishments need to invest in training and equipment.

3. Resistance to change

- **Job concerns**: Fear that technology will replace human labor.
- **Established habits** : Difficulty in changing entrenched practices.

4. Ethical and legal issues

- **Data protection**: Respect the confidentiality and security of information collected.
- **Professional responsibility**: Understand the legal implications of using technology.

Strategies for effective training

1. Progressive and adapted approach

- **Modular training**: divide training into short modules to facilitate learning.
- **Hands-on learning**: workshops and demonstrations in real-life situations.

2. Institutional support

- **Ongoing training programs**: Establishments must offer regular training as part of their work schedule.

- ○ **Personalized support**: Tutors or mentors are available to help caregivers with their apprenticeship.

3. Use of digital resources

- ○ **E-learning**: Online courses accessible at any time, allowing you to adapt to your own pace.
- ○ **Communities of practice**: Forums, online groups for exchanging with peers and sharing experiences.

4. Valuing acquired skills

- ○ **Professional recognition**: Certificates, validation of prior learning to motivate care assistants.
- ○ **Development prospects**: Opportunities for career advancement thanks to new skills.

5. Integrating ethics and legislation into training

- ○ **Raising awareness of issues**: Addressing questions of confidentiality, consent and responsibility.
- ○ **Regulatory update**: Inform on current laws and regulations concerning medical technologies.

The positive impact on daily practice

1. Efficiency gains

- ○ **Automate repetitive tasks**: Reduce time spent on administrative tasks.
- ○ **Better organization**: optimized care planning thanks to digital tools.

2. Improved communication

- ○ **Easier exchanges**: instant communication with the care team, real-time information sharing.

184

- ○ **Traceability of actions**: History of care provided, tracking of interventions.

3. Enhanced patient safety

- ○ **Error reduction**: Alerts in case of incorrect dosage, drug incompatibilities.
- ○ **Increased surveillance**: Early detection of anomalies thanks to monitoring devices.

4. Increased job satisfaction

- ○ **Sense of competence**: Mastering new technologies boosts self-confidence.
- ○ **Role recognition**: Visible contribution to innovation and improved care.

Concrete examples of successful integration

1. Using tablets for care
The nursing auxiliary uses a tablet to access patient files, record the care provided and consult protocols. This enables real-time updating of information, reduces transcription errors, and improves coordination with the team.

2. Virtual reality training
Virtual reality training sessions enable caregivers to practice technical gestures in a simulated environment, without risk to patients. This improves their mastery of gestures and boosts confidence before putting them into practice.

3. Remote monitoring of vital signs
Thanks to connected devices, caregivers can continuously monitor patients' vital parameters, even when they are not physically present at their side. In the event of an anomaly, an alert is triggered, enabling rapid intervention.

- Security and confidentiality of patient data

The security and confidentiality of patient data are crucial issues in the healthcare sector. With the increasing digitization of medical information, the protection of personal data has become a major concern for healthcare professionals, care facilities and patients themselves. In Internal Medicine, where sensitive information is frequently handled, it is essential to understand the legal, ethical and practical obligations associated with data management. This chapter explores the importance of patient data security and confidentiality, the responsibilities of caregivers, good practice and current challenges in this area.

The importance of patient data security and confidentiality

1. **Respect for fundamental rights**

   The right to privacy and protection of personal data is a fundamental right recognized by the Universal Declaration of Human Rights and national legislation. Patients have the right to control who has access to their medical information and how it is used.

2. **Trust between patient and healthcare professional**

   A relationship of trust is at the heart of medical practice. Patients must be able to confide fully in their caregivers, knowing that their information will be treated with discretion and respect. Guaranteed confidentiality encourages open communication, which is essential for effective care.

3. **Preventing harm**

   Unauthorized disclosure of medical data can lead to negative consequences for patients, such as discrimination, stigmatization or impacts on their personal and professional lives. Data security aims to prevent these risks.

Legal and regulatory framework

1. **The General Data Protection Regulation (GDPR)**
   Coming into force in May 2018, the RGPD strengthens the protection of personal data within the European Union. It imposes strict obligations on organizations that process data, including healthcare establishments, concerning the collection, processing, storage and security of information.

2. **The French Public Health Code**
   In France, the Code de la Santé Publique stipulates that healthcare professionals are bound by medical secrecy. Any breach is liable to penal and disciplinary sanctions.

3. **CNIL recommendations**
   The Commission Nationale de l'Informatique et des Libertés (CNIL) issues specific recommendations for the healthcare sector, guiding data protection practices.

The caregiver's role and responsibilities

1. **Professional secrecy**
   Like all other healthcare professionals, nursing auxiliaries are bound by professional secrecy. They must take care not to divulge any information that comes to their knowledge in the course of their duties, whether verbally, in writing or by any other means.

2. **Information management**

   - **Limited access to data**: Access only to the information needed to carry out your tasks.
   - **Secure transmission**: Share information with the healthcare team only if it is relevant to the patient's care, using secure channels.
   - **Discretion**: Avoid discussing patients in public places or in the presence of unauthorized persons.

3. **Use of digital tools**

With the digitization of patient records, the nursing auxiliary must :

- ○ **Log in with personal identifiers**: Do not share your access codes.
- ○ **Close sessions after use**: prevent unauthorized access to information.
- ○ **Report anomalies**: Inform the IT department in the event of a suspected security breach or malfunction.

Best practices for data security

1. **Training and awareness-raising**

- ○ **Participate in training**: Keep abreast of security protocols, legislative updates and new threats.
- ○ **Understand the risks**: be aware of the possible consequences of a data breach for the patient and the establishment.

2. **Adopt a proactive attitude**

- ○ **Verify identity**: Before transmitting any information, make sure that the person you are communicating with is who you say he or she is, and that he or she has the right to access the data.
- ○ **Use strong passwords**: Choose complex passwords and change them regularly.
- ○ **Avoid unsecured media**: Do not store patient information on unprotected personal devices (USB sticks, personal computers).

3. Secure communication

- ○ **Avoid sensitive conversations in public**: Do not discuss patient cases in corridors, elevators or other places where third parties may overhear.
- ○ **Use institutional tools**: Give preference to secure messaging systems provided by the establishment for all professional communication.

Current challenges and possible solutions

1. Cyber threats
Healthcare facilities are targets for cyberattacks, such as ransomware, which can compromise patient data.

- ○ **Solutions** :
  - ▪ **Regular updates**: Ensure that systems and software are up to date to benefit from the latest protection.
  - ▪ **Enhanced security**: Use antivirus, firewall and intrusion detection systems.

2. Multiplying data access points
With the development of telemedicine and healthcare applications, data access points are multiplying.

- ○ **Solutions** :
  - ▪ **Access control**: Implement strong authentication policies.
  - ▪ **Traceability**: Record data access to detect any anomalies.

3. Balancing accessibility and security
Facilitating access to information for rapid care while protecting data is a constant challenge.

- ◦ **Solutions** :
  - ▪ **Clear policies**: Define protocols that reconcile effective care and data protection.
  - ▪ **Ongoing training**: Raising staff awareness of best practices, so that they become active players in safety.

Case studies illustrating safety principles

1. **Situation: Using a shared computer workstation**
    The orderly uses a computer to consult a patient's file. After his consultation, he is called in an emergency and leaves the workstation without disconnecting.

    - ◦ **Risk**: Unauthorized access to data.
    - ◦ **Best practice**: Always lock or log off before leaving your workstation, even for a short absence.

2. **Situation: Request for information by telephone**
    A caller introduces himself as a family member and asks for information about a patient's state of health.

    - ◦ **Risk**: Disclosure of information to an unauthorized person.
    - ◦ **Best practice**: Do not give out sensitive information over the telephone unless you are sure of the caller's identity and right to receive the information. Refer the caller to the appropriate doctor or service.

The role of technology in data security

1. **Data encryption**
    Sensitive data must be encrypted, both at rest and during transmission, to prevent unauthorized access.

2. **Multi-factor authentication**

   The use of multiple authentication methods (password, badge, fingerprint) enhances system access security.

3. **Identity management software**

   These tools enable you to manage access rights according to each user's role, thus limiting data exposure.

Responsibilities in the event of a data breach

1. **Legal obligations**

   In the event of a breach, the establishment must notify the CNIL and, in some cases, the patients concerned. Penalties may include substantial fines.

2. **Professional consequences**

   Staff involved in a violation may be subject to disciplinary or even criminal sanctions, depending on the seriousness of the misconduct.

3. **Impact on reputation**

   A data breach can damage patient confidence and affect the reputation of the facility.

Chapter 9

Case studies and practical examples

- Analysis of complex clinical situations

The practice of the internal medicine orderly is often confronted with complex clinical situations requiring in-depth analysis, critical reflection and constant adaptation. These situations may arise from the severity of pathologies, the multiplicity of health problems within a single patient, or the interactions between the physical, psychological and social aspects of illness. The nursing auxiliary plays a key role in analyzing these situations, in close collaboration with the care team, to ensure effective, comprehensive patient care. This chapter explores the importance of analyzing complex clinical situations, the skills required to deal with them, and strategies for optimizing caregiving intervention in these contexts.

Understanding complexity in internal medicine

Internal medicine is a discipline characterized by the management of patients with multiple, often chronic and interconnected pathologies. Clinical complexity stems from several factors:

1. **Pluripathology**: Patients may suffer from several diseases simultaneously, such as diabetes, heart failure and kidney disease, complicating diagnosis, treatment and follow-up.

2. **Polymedication**: The use of multiple medications increases the risk of drug interactions, side effects and poor compliance.

3. **Advanced age and frailty**: Elderly patients often have diminished physiological reserves, increased vulnerability to stress, and specific care needs.

4. **Psychosocial factors**: Social situation, family support, cultural beliefs and psychological factors influence the way patients experience their illness and adhere to treatment.

The caregiver's role in analyzing complex situations

The caregiver is close to the patient, in a privileged position to observe, understand and intervene in complex situations. Responsibilities include :

1. Fine, systematic observation

- **Clinical signs**: Note changes in the patient's general condition, such as temperature, pain, breathing, appetite, sleep.
- **Behavior and mood**: Watch for signs of depression, anxiety, agitation or confusion.
- **Daily functioning**: Assess the patient's autonomy in activities of daily living, such as hygiene, eating and mobility.

2. Patient communication

- **Active listening**: Allowing patients to express their concerns, symptoms and difficulties.
- **Empathy and support**: Creating a climate of trust to facilitate the sharing of sensitive information.

3. Collaboration with the care team

- **Transmitting information**: Clearly and accurately communicate observations to nurses and doctors.
- **Participation in summary meetings**: Contribute to the development of the care plan by sharing your point of view.
- **Coordination of interventions**: Collaborate with different professionals (physiotherapist, dietician, psychologist) for a multidisciplinary approach.

Skills for analyzing complex situations

1. **In-depth knowledge**

   ○ **Common pathologies in internal medicine**: Understanding the signs, symptoms and specific needs associated with the main diseases.
   ○ **Basic pharmacology**: Learn about the effects of commonly used drugs, and the signs of side effects or toxicity.

2. **Observation and evaluation skills**

   ○ **Detailed observation**: Develop a keen sense of observation to detect subtle changes.
   ○ **Critical analysis**: Relate observations to knowledge to identify potential problems.

3. **Effective communication**

   ○ **Clarity and precision**: Convey information concisely, using appropriate language.
   ○ **Adapting to the patient** : Adapt communication to the patient's cognitive, cultural and linguistic abilities.

4. **Ethical reflection**

   ○ **Respect for autonomy**: Consider patient choices and preferences when planning care.
   ○ **Confidentiality**: Protect sensitive information while ensuring effective communication with the team.

Strategies for intervention in complex situations

1. **Patient-centered approach**

   ○ **Personalized care**: Adapting interventions to the patient's specific needs, taking into account his or her preferences, values and life context.
   ○ **Active patient participation**: Encourage patients to get involved in decisions concerning their health.

2. **Interdisciplinary teamwork**

   ○ **Coordination**: working with different professionals to ensure coherent, integrated care.
   ○ **Sharing information**: Use effective communication tools, such as shared files, team meetings and written transmissions.

3. **Planning and prioritization**

   ○ **Identify key problems**: Assess priorities according to severity, urgency and impact on quality of life.
   ○ **Structured action plan**: Establish clear objectives, specific interventions and evaluation criteria.

4. **Continuing education**

   ○ **Updating knowledge**: Participate in training courses, workshops and readings to keep abreast of medical advances and best practices.
   ○ **Reflecting on practice**: Analyze situations encountered, identify lessons learned, and adjust future approaches.

Examples of complex clinical situations

1. Elderly polymorbid patient with acute confusion

- **Background**: Mr Martin, 82, hospitalized with pneumonia, also had heart failure and diabetes. He suddenly develops confusion, with nocturnal agitation.
- **Caregiver intervention**:
  - **Observation**: Note signs of disorientation, changes in behavior, diuresis, blood glucose.
  - **Communication**: Inform nurse of observations, participate in delirium risk assessment.
  - **Specific actions**: Ensure a calm environment, secure the patient to prevent falls, promote orientation in time and place (clock, calendar).
  - **Collaboration**: Working with the team to adjust the care plan, e.g. adapting sleep schedules, pain management.

2. Patients with chronic wounds and malnutrition

- **Background**: Mrs Dupont, 65, suffers from leg ulcers linked to venous insufficiency, and is malnourished due to anorexia.
- **Caregiver intervention**:
  - **Observation**: Monitor wound condition, food intake, weight, signs of infection.
  - **Nutritional support**: Encourage eating habits, offer protein-rich snacks, work with the dietician.
  - **Local care**: Participate in hygiene care to preserve skin integrity, apply pressure sore prevention protocols.

- **Education**: Inform the patient about the importance of nutrition for healing, support motivation.

Managing the challenges of complex situations

1. Emotional charge

- **Recognizing emotions**: Be aware of the emotional impact these situations can have on the caregiver.
- **Professional support**: Participate in discussion groups, share with colleagues, seek help from the team psychologist.

2. Time management

- **Organization**: Plan tasks according to priorities, use time management tools.
- **Asking for help**: Don't hesitate to ask for support from colleagues or management in case of overload.

3. Communications complexity

- **Adaptation**: Use communication techniques adapted to patients with cognitive or linguistic difficulties.
- **Training**: Training in alternative communication methods, such as non-verbal communication and visual aids.

The importance of ethical reflection

In complex situations, ethical dilemmas may arise:

- **Autonomy vs. safety**: Respecting a patient's wish to go home despite risks.
- **Confidentiality vs. the need to share information**: Communicating sensitive information for the good of the patient.

The orderly must :

- **Reflect on the values at stake**: Identify the ethical principles involved.
- **Consult the team**: Discuss dilemmas with colleagues, manager, ethics committee if necessary.
- **Make informed decisions**: Act with respect for the patient and professional obligations.

- Handling contingencies and emergencies

Dealing with the unexpected and emergencies is an essential part of the role of the internal medicine orderly. Emergencies can arise at any time, and the orderly, as front-line patient carer, must be able to react quickly and effectively. This ability to deal with the unexpected relies on a combination of knowledge, practical skills, professional attitudes and collaboration with the nursing team. This chapter explores the fundamentals of contingency and emergency management, the skills required, the protocols to follow, and the importance of preparation and ongoing training.

Understanding contingencies and emergencies in internal medicine

In Internal Medicine, patients often present with complex and unstable pathologies, increasing the risk of sudden complications. The unexpected can include:

1. **Sudden deterioration in health**: drop in blood pressure, respiratory distress, heart rhythm disorders.
2. **Acute events**: angina pectoris, stroke, digestive haemorrhage.
3. **Adverse reactions to treatment**: Drug allergies, serious side effects.
4. **Accidents** : Falls, injuries, ingestion of harmful substances.

The ability to recognize these situations quickly and act appropriately is crucial to patient safety and prognosis.

The caregiver's role in emergency management

1. **Observation and early detection**

    o   **Constant vigilance**: Be attentive to the patient's vital signs, physical appearance, behavior and complaints.
    o   **Recognizing warning signs**: Identify symptoms that indicate an emergency, such as chest pain, dyspnea, sudden confusion, bleeding.

2. **Immediate reaction**

    o   **Alert the nursing team**: Immediately inform the nurse or doctor in the event of a critical situation, providing precise, concise information.
    o   **Introduction to first aid**: If trained and authorized, begin first aid procedures such as cardiopulmonary resuscitation (CPR), placing the patient in the lateral position of safety and compressing a bleed.

3. **Application of emergency protocols**

    o   **Knowledge of procedures**: Master internal protocols for specific emergency situations.
    o   **Use of emergency equipment**: Know where to find emergency equipment (defibrillator, emergency cart) and how to use it.

4. **Assistance to the medical team**

    o   **Material preparation**: Bring in the necessary materials, prepare the equipment, install the patient as indicated.
    o   **Active collaboration**: Follow the nurse's or doctor's instructions, participate in maneuvers if necessary.

5. **Patient and family support**

   ○ **Communication**: Reassure the patient if possible, calmly explain what is happening.
   ○ **Dealing with loved ones**: Inform them with empathy, guide them to an appropriate waiting area.

Emergency management skills

1. **Theoretical knowledge**

   ○ **Physiopathology**: Understanding the mechanisms of common internal medicine emergencies.
   ○ **First aid**: Learn basic first aid and resuscitation techniques.

2. **Practical skills**

   ○ **CPR technique**: Learn how to perform effective chest compressions and insufflations.
   ○ **Use of the automated external defibrillator (AED)**: Be trained in its use.

3. **Non-technical skills**

   ○ **Stress management**: Staying calm, making quick, rational decisions.
   ○ **Effective communication**: convey information clearly, listen to instructions.

4. **Professional attitudes**

   ○ **Proactivity**: Don't hesitate to act in the patient's best interest.
   ○ **Team spirit**: work in harmony with colleagues, support team effort.

Emergency protocols and procedures

1. **Alarm and resource mobilization**

    ○ **Alert procedures**: Know internal call numbers, emergency codes (e.g. "Code Bleu").
    ○ **Team mobilization**: Ensure that all necessary stakeholders are informed.

2. **Patient and environmental safety**

    ○ **Scene assessment**: Check that the environment is safe for the patient and caregivers.
    ○ **Preventing complications**: For example, clear the airway, avoid unnecessary movements in case of trauma.

3. **Documentation and traceability**

    ○ **Record events**: Note times, actions taken, important observations.
    ○ **Communication with the relevant departments**: If necessary, prepare for transfer to an intensive care unit or specialized service.

Training and preparation

1. **Initial and continuing training**

    ○ **Certifications**: Obtain and keep up to date first aid and CPR certifications.
    ○ **Internal training**: Participate in training sessions organized by the company.

2. **Simulations and practical exercises**

    ○ **Emergency scenarios**: Take part in simulations to reinforce reflexes and coordination.
    ○ **Debriefings**: After exercises or real emergencies, analyze actions to learn from them.

3. Knowledge of equipment

- ○ **Equipment location**: Know where to find emergency carts, defibrillators and oxygen therapy equipment.
- ○ **Handling equipment**: Practice using devices so you're ready when you need to be.

Managing non-medical contingencies

The unexpected is not just a medical emergency. The caregiver may be confronted with other unforeseen situations:

1. Staff absences

- ○ **Reorganizing work**: adapting task allocation, prioritizing essential care.
- ○ **Communication**: Inform the health executive, ask for back-up if necessary.

2. Equipment failure

- ○ **Report**: Immediately inform the technical department.
- ○ **Alternative solutions**: Use replacement equipment, adapt work methods.

3. Environmental incidents

- ○ **Fires, floods, power cuts**: Learn about evacuation plans and emergency procedures.
- ○ **Ensure patient safety**: Assist with evacuation, maintain comfort and safety.

Emotional impact and support

1. Managing emotions

- **Awareness**: Recognize your own reactions to stress and critical situations.
- **Coping techniques**: Using methods to manage stress, such as deep breathing and positive thinking.

2. Mutual support

- **Team debriefing**: sharing experiences, expressing emotions, supporting colleagues.
- **Access to resources**: Seek help from a psychologist or support professional if necessary.

3. Burn-out prevention

- **Work-life balance**: Make sure you get enough rest and maintain pleasant activities outside work.
- **Stress management training**: Participate in workshops or training courses to develop resilience skills.

Case study: Reacting to sudden deterioration

Mrs Lefèvre, aged 68, hospitalized for renal failure, suddenly complains of chest pain and develops dyspnoea.

- **Caregiver's observation**: Notes sudden onset of symptoms, pale face, cold sweat.
- **Immediate action**:
  - **Alert**: Quickly informs the nurse with precise details.
  - **Positioning**: Help the patient to sit up to facilitate breathing.
  - **Measure vital signs**: If possible, take blood pressure, pulse, oxygen saturation.

- **Team support** :
  - ° **Equipment preparation**: Bring emergency cart, prepare oxygen.
  - ° **Patient support**: Stay with her, reassure her, monitor the evolution of her symptoms.

- Problem-solving strategies

Effective problem-solving is a fundamental skill for the internal medicine orderly. Faced with varied and often complex situations, the orderly must be able to analyze challenges, propose appropriate solutions and implement suitable actions to ensure patients' well-being. This chapter explores the different problem-solving strategies, the key stages in the process, the skills required and the importance of inter-professional collaboration in developing effective solutions.

Understanding the nature of problems in internal medicine

In internal medicine, the problems encountered by the orderly can be of various kinds:

1. **Clinical issues**: Managing symptoms, observing signs of deterioration, adapting care to specific patient needs.

2. **Organizational issues**: Care planning, time management, coordination with the nursing team, availability of equipment.

3. **Relational issues**: communication with patients and their families, conflict management, adapting to cultural and linguistic diversity.

4. **Ethical issues**: Dilemmas linked to respect for patient autonomy, confidentiality, end-of-life decisions.

Key problem-solving steps

1. **Identifying the problem**

   - **Careful observation**: become aware of the problematic situation through careful observation of the facts.

   - **Precise definition**: Clearly formulate the problem in specific, understandable terms.

2. **Problem analysis**

   - **Information gathering**: Gather all relevant data, including patient history, clinical observations and contextual information.

   - **Understanding causes**: Identifying contributing factors, distinguishing root causes from apparent symptoms.

3. **Generating possible solutions**

   - **Brainstorming**: Propose various options without initial judgment, encourage creativity.

   - **Consultation**: Involve colleagues, nurses and doctors to benefit from multiple perspectives.

4. **Evaluating options**

   - **Analysis of advantages and disadvantages**: Consider the potential effectiveness, feasibility and risks associated with each solution.

   - **Taking resources into account**: Evaluate the availability of materials, time and personnel.

5. Choosing the best solution

- ○ **Informed decision**: Select the most appropriate option based on the previous analysis.

- ○ **Validation with the team**: Confirm the choice with colleagues and superiors if necessary.

6. Solution implementation

- ○ **Action plan**: Define precise stages, responsibilities and deadlines.

- ○ **Communication**: Inform all parties involved, including the patient if relevant.

7. Evaluation of results

- ○ **Follow-up**: Observe the effects of the solution implemented, gather feedback.

- ○ **Adjustment** : Make modifications if necessary, learn from experience for future situations.

Skills for effective problem solving

1. Critical thinking

- ○ **Logical analysis**: The ability to evaluate information rationally and objectively.

- ○ **Ability to synthesize**: integrate different sources of information to get a global view.

2. Creativity

- ○ **Innovation**: proposing original solutions when traditional approaches fail.

- ○ **Flexibility**: Adapt to changing situations, open to new ideas.

3. Effective communication

- ○ **Active listening**: Understanding the needs and concerns of patients and colleagues.

- ○ **Clarity of expression**: Explain problems and solutions in an understandable way.

4. Stress management

- ○ **Calm under pressure**: maintain composure in urgent or difficult situations.

- ○ **Resilience**: The ability to bounce back from obstacles and setbacks.

5. Teamwork

- ○ **Collaboration**: working in harmony with other professionals, sharing responsibilities.

- ○ **Mutual respect**: Valuing each other's contributions, fostering a climate of trust.

Specific problem-solving strategies

1. Systematic approach

- ○ **Use of models**: Apply problem-solving frameworks such as DESC (Describe, Express, Specify, Conclude) to structure thinking.

- ◦ **Institutional protocols**: Refer to established procedures to guide actions.

2. **Prioritization**

   - ◦ **Urgency assessment**: Determine which problems require immediate attention.

   - ◦ **Time management**: allocate resources efficiently, avoid dispersion.

3. **Search for resources**

   - ◦ **Documentation**: Consult clinical guidelines, manuals and medical databases.

   - ◦ **Expert consultation**: Call on specialists or experienced colleagues for advice.

4. **Ethical reflection**

   - ◦ **Consideration of values**: Take into account ethical principles, patient rights and legal obligations.

   - ◦ **Moral dilemmas**: Analyze complex situations where solutions may have contradictory consequences.

Examples of situations and practical applications

1. **Managing unrelieved pain**

   - ◦ **Identification**: A patient complains of persistent pain despite ongoing treatment.

   - ◦ **Analysis**: Check correct administration of analgesics, observe associated signs, assess pain intensity.

- ○ **Possible solutions**: Suggest a medical re-evaluation, consider non-pharmacological techniques (relaxation, repositioning), check for possible side effects or drug tolerance.

- ○ **Implementation**: Inform nurse, apply appropriate interventions, monitor patient response.

2. **Preventing falls in at-risk patients**

- ○ **Identification**: An elderly patient presents with balance problems and a history of falls.

- ○ **Analysis**: Assess environment (slippery floors, obstacles), personal factors (muscle weakness, confusion), medications that may affect balance.

- ○ **Possible solutions**: Install technical aids (grab bars, light path), adjust care plan for increased monitoring, coordinate with physiotherapist for strengthening exercises.

- ○ **Implementation**: Implement measures, inform the team, educate the patient on precautions to be taken.

Importance of reflection on practice

- • **Self-evaluation**: After solving a problem, reflect on the process, identifying what went well and what could be improved.

- • **Continuous learning**: Use every situation as a learning opportunity, share experiences with colleagues.

- • **Professional development**: Participate in training courses, workshops and discussion groups to deepen problem-solving skills.

The role of technology in problem solving

- **Digital tools**: Use applications and software to quickly access information, follow protocols and communicate with the team.

- **Medical databases**: search for up-to-date information on pathologies, treatments and drug interactions.

- **Simulations and online training**: practice solving complex clinical situations through interactive scenarios.

Interprofessional collaboration

- **Synergy of skills**: Take advantage of complementary expertise within the team (nurses, doctors, therapists).

- **Interdisciplinary communication**: Participate in department meetings, briefings and debriefings to align approaches.

- **Respecting roles**: understanding the limits of your field of action, knowing when to delegate or ask for help.

- Feedback and lessons learned

In the field of internal medicine, the nursing auxiliary plays a central role in the overall care of patients. Beyond technical skills and medical knowledge, continuous learning through feedback is essential to improve the quality of care, reinforce professional practices and foster personal development. This chapter explores the importance of feedback, how it enriches the caregiver's practice, how to integrate it effectively, and the valuable lessons that can be learned from it.

The importance of feedback in healthcare practice

Feedback is a reflexive process that enables us to learn from both positive and negative situations. It provides an opportunity to :

1. **Improving professional skills**: By analyzing the actions undertaken and their results, the orderly identifies the strong points to be reinforced and the areas for improvement.

2. **Preventing errors**: Understanding the causes of incidents or errors enables preventive measures to be put in place to avoid their recurrence.

3. **Encourage collective learning**: sharing experiences with colleagues enriches the team's knowledge, encourages collaboration and strengthens cohesion.

4. **Enhancing the quality of care**: By integrating the lessons learned, the caregiver contributes to more effective, safe care adapted to patients' needs.

Integrating feedback into daily practice

1. **Systematic self-reflection**
   Caregivers are encouraged to adopt a regular reflective approach:

   - **After each significant situation,** take time to reflect on the actions taken, the decisions made and their consequences.

   - **Identify successes**: Acknowledging what has worked well boosts self-confidence and encourages the replication of these practices.

   - **Analyze difficulties**: Understand the obstacles encountered, the mistakes made and the contributing factors.

2. **Participation in department meetings**
Team meetings provide an ideal setting for sharing experiences:

- ○ **Present clinical cases**: Discuss complex or unusual situations to benefit from colleagues' perspectives.

- ○ **Debrief incidents**: Collectively analyze undesirable events to identify root causes and develop solutions.

- ○ **Exchange best practices**: share effective methods, tips and innovations.

3. **Use of monitoring and evaluation tools**

- ○ **Logbooks**: Keep a logbook to record significant experiences, reflections and learning.

- ○ **Self-assessment grids**: Use tools to assess skills and monitor progress.

- ○ **Formalized feedback**: Solicit feedback from colleagues, nurses or healthcare managers.

Lessons learned: concrete examples

1. **Improved communication with patients**
When a patient expresses confusion or anxiety about a treatment, the caregiver realizes that the language used was too technical. By adapting his or her discourse, using simple terms and checking the patient's understanding, he or she finds that the patient is more cooperative and calmer.

2. **Managing an aggressive situation**
Confronted with an agitated patient, the caregiver initially reacts with an authoritarian attitude, exacerbating the

tension. After reflection, he or she understands the importance of empathic listening and verbal de-escalation. In a similar situation later, he adopts a calm approach, shows understanding, and succeeds in calming the patient.

3. Preventing medication errors
After observing a mix-up between two patients with similar names, the orderly realizes the crucial importance of systematically checking the patient's identity before any treatment. This experience leads to increased vigilance and the promotion of this practice among the team.

Factors facilitating learning from experience

1. Open-mindedness and humility
Recognizing that you can always learn and improve is essential. Caregivers must be ready to accept constructive criticism and question their practices.

2. A caring environment
A climate of trust within the team encourages the sharing of experiences without fear of judgment. Mistakes are seen as learning opportunities rather than failures.

3. Institutional support
Healthcare establishments that value continuing education, provide forums for discussion and encourage a quality approach facilitate the integration of lessons learned.

Challenges in applying lessons learned

1. Resistance to change
Changing ingrained habits can be difficult. It's important to understand the obstacles to change and address them appropriately.

2. **High workload**
Lack of time can limit reflection and the sharing of experiences. It's crucial to set aside time for these activities, even in busy schedules.

3. **Lack of recognition**
If efforts to improve are not recognized, this can demotivate caregivers. A culture of valuing positive initiatives is beneficial.

Strategies for overcoming obstacles

1. **Integrating feedback into the routine**

   ○ **Plan regular moments**: For example, set up a short debriefing at the end of the day or shift.

   ○ **Use technology**: Online platforms, internal forums to quickly share experiences and ideas.

2. **Encouraging group training**

   ○ **Hands-on workshops**: Participate in interactive training courses where experiences are shared.

   ○ **Support groups**: Create peer groups to discuss challenges and solutions.

3. **Promoting collaborative leadership**

   ○ **Involve healthcare managers**: Their support is essential to creating a learning culture.

   ○ **Valuing initiatives**: Publicly recognize the contributions of caregivers who share their experiences and suggest improvements.

The impact of lessons learned on quality of care

1. **Enhancing professional skills**
   Continuous learning leads to better mastery of techniques, faster adaptation to new situations and more informed decision-making.

2. **Improving patient safety**
   By learning from past mistakes, caregivers help reduce the risk of incidents and increase the reliability of care.

3. **Increased patient satisfaction**
   Better care, effective communication and an empathetic attitude improve the patient experience and boost confidence.

4. **Professional fulfillment**
   Feeling like you're making progress, adding value and being recognized for your efforts contributes to job satisfaction and motivation.

Chapter 10

Conclusion

- The impact of the orderly in Internal Medicine

Nurses play a fundamental role in Internal Medicine departments. On the front line of care, they are the essential link between the patient and the medical team. Their role goes far beyond the simple execution of practical tasks; they are at the heart of human support, quality of care and the department's operational efficiency. This impact, although sometimes discreet, is deeply felt by patients, families and healthcare professionals alike. This chapter explores in depth the decisive influence of the nursing auxiliary in Internal Medicine, highlighting the many facets of its daily commitment.

Contributing to quality of care

The nursing auxiliary is the guarantor of the basic care that is essential to the well-being of patients. They ensure personal hygiene, help with feeding, mobilization and comfort, all of which are fundamental to the dignity and health of hospitalized patients. Through their attentive presence, they detect subtle clinical signs that may indicate a deteriorating state of health: suspicious redness, a change in appetite, discreetly expressed pain. These observations are crucial and are passed on to the nursing or medical team, enabling rapid and appropriate intervention. In this way, the caregiver contributes directly to the prevention of complications, clinical monitoring and treatment efficacy.

Emotional and psychosocial support

In addition to physical care, the nursing auxiliary plays an essential role in providing emotional support to patients. Internal Medicine often cares for people with chronic, complex or serious illnesses, generating stress, anxiety and uncertainty. The caregiver is an attentive ear, offering a reassuring and empathetic presence. They take the time to listen to concerns, answer questions, share a kind word or a smile that can brighten a patient's day. This human accompaniment promotes psychological well-being, boosts morale and can even have a positive impact on recovery. By supporting families too, the caregiver helps to create an environment of trust and serenity around the patient.

Interprofessional collaboration

Effective care in internal medicine depends on close collaboration between the various healthcare professionals. The nursing auxiliary is an active member of this multidisciplinary team. They communicate regularly with nurses, doctors, physiotherapists, dieticians and social workers, sharing their observations and contributing to an overall understanding of the patient's situation. Her detailed knowledge of patients' daily needs and reactions enriches clinical decisions. This collaboration promotes coherent, coordinated, patient-centred care, improving clinical outcomes and patient satisfaction.

Improving patient satisfaction

The patient experience is a key indicator of quality of care. The caregiver's proximity and availability play a decisive role in the patient's perception of his or her hospital stay. By personalizing care, respecting individual preferences and demonstrating patience and understanding, they help to create a warm and respectful atmosphere. Patients feel listened to, valued and supported, reducing stress and anxiety. This special attention can transform a potentially trying experience into a positive and reassuring care journey.

Contributing to operational efficiency

The orderly plays an active role in the organization and efficiency of the Internal Medicine department. By effectively managing their time, prioritizing tasks and optimizing the use of resources, they support the smooth running of the department. He/she ensures compliance with protocols and procedures, prevents errors and incidents, and participates in the training of new staff members. This helps to reduce delays, improve care coordination and ensure patient safety. In addition, by alerting the care team quickly to any problems, he or she helps avoid complications and facilitates early intervention.

Role in health education

Nurses also play an important role in patient education. They inform them about the care they are receiving, and guide them in learning gestures that promote their autonomy, such as mobilization or breathing exercises. They encourage healthy behavior, raise awareness of hygiene measures, and prepare patients for their return home in collaboration with the nursing team. This educational support reinforces patient autonomy, encourages compliance with treatment and helps prevent re-hospitalization.

Impact on the prevention of nosocomial infections

Preventing healthcare-associated infections is a major challenge in the hospital environment. By strictly adhering to hygiene measures such as hand washing, the use of personal protective equipment and surface disinfection, orderlies play a key role in reducing the risk of infection. They also make patients and visitors aware of the precautions to be taken, thereby helping to protect everyone.

Promoting a culture of caring and respect

The caregiver's attitude influences the climate of the department. By showing respect, tolerance and open-mindedness, they help to create an environment where everyone feels accepted and valued. This culture of caring promotes staff well-being, reduces stress, and has a positive impact on the quality of interactions with patients. It also encourages collaboration and solidarity within the team, boosting collective efficiency.

Contribution to training and innovation

The nursing auxiliary participates in the training of students and new colleagues, sharing its experience and knowledge. They are often involved in quality improvement projects, putting forward ideas to optimize practices, improve patient comfort or enhance care safety. His involvement in innovation reflects his commitment to excellence and the positive evolution of the profession.

Role in managing end-of-life situations

In internal medicine, the nursing auxiliary is sometimes called upon to accompany patients at the end of life. Their role is crucial in ensuring the comfort, dignity and emotional support of patients and their families. Through their discreet, attentive presence, they bring an essential human dimension to these delicate moments, contributing to quality palliative care.

- Incentives for future professionals

The profession of internal medicine orderly is much more than a job; it's a vocation, a commitment to people, a passion for caring and supporting those who need it most. To all you future professionals preparing to embrace this noble career, I offer this encouragement to light your way and strengthen your resolve.

The importance of your role

From the moment you enter this field, you'll realize just how essential your role is. You will be the guardians of comfort, the sentinels of well-being and the artisans of patient dignity. Every gesture you make will have a profound impact on the lives of those you accompany. Your presence, your words, your attentiveness will have the power to comfort, restore hope and relieve suffering. Never forget that, although sometimes discreet, your impact is immense and precious.

Cultivating compassion and empathy

Internal Medicine will bring you face to face with complex situations, heavy pathologies and sometimes difficult life paths. In the face of these challenges, it's your compassion that will make the difference. Cultivate the ability to put yourself in the other person's shoes, to understand their fears, doubts and hopes. Empathy will be your compass, guiding your actions and enriching your relationships with patients and their families. By being attentive to each person's needs, you'll provide genuine and profound support.

Developing your skills

Technical know-how is indispensable, but it must be constantly nurtured and renewed. Be curious, invest in your training, seek out learning opportunities. Medical and technological advances evolve rapidly, and your willingness to learn will enable you to stay at the cutting edge, offer quality care and develop professionally. Don't hesitate to ask questions, take part in ongoing training and share your knowledge with colleagues.

The importance of teamwork

You'll never be alone in your missions. The strength of Internal Medicine lies in inter-professional collaboration. Enjoy the richness of exchanges with nurses, doctors, physiotherapists and all other healthcare professionals. Everyone makes their own contribution, and together you can offer the best possible care to your patients. Promote communication, mutual respect and solidarity within the team. These enriching professional relationships will contribute to your personal development and the effectiveness of your care.

Facing challenges with resilience

The road ahead won't always be easy. You'll be faced with challenging situations, moments of doubt and intense emotions. It's important to recognize these feelings, take care of yourself and develop your resilience. Learn to manage stress, find a balance between your professional and personal life, and seek support when you need it. Your well-being is essential if you are to support others with kindness and energy.

Keeping a sense of commitment

When you feel tired or discouraged, remember the reasons that led you to choose this profession. The desire to help, a passion for caring and the pleasure of creating meaningful human relationships are the driving forces that will carry you through your career. Every smile, every sincere thank-you, every patient improvement will be rewards that give meaning to your commitment.

Being an agent of change

The healthcare system is constantly evolving, and you have a role to play in this dynamic. Don't hesitate to share your ideas, suggest improvements and take part in projects aimed at optimizing practices. Your insight is invaluable, and your experience in the field brings added value to our collective thinking. By being proactive, you'll be helping to shape an Internal Medicine that's more efficient, more humane and better adapted to patients' needs.

Celebrate your successes

Take the time to recognize your accomplishments, even the smallest ones. Every challenge overcome, every skill acquired, every relationship of trust established is a victory. These successes mark out your career path and build your professional identity. They reflect your commitment, perseverance and talent. Be proud of how far you've come, and let that pride fuel your motivation for the challenges ahead.

- The future of the nursing profession

Caregivers have long held a central position in the healthcare system, providing essential care and close support to patients. At the dawn of the XXIe century, the profession finds itself at a decisive turning point, facing major challenges but also bringing unprecedented opportunities. Demographic change, technological advances, societal mutations and transformations in the healthcare system are redrawing the contours of the profession. This chapter explores the future of the nursing profession, highlighting emerging trends, crucial issues and prospects for those who embrace this vocation.

Growing demand for personalized care

The aging of the population is one of the most striking phenomena of our time. Increased life expectancy, coupled with the growing prevalence of chronic illnesses, is generating a growing demand for long-term care and personalized support. Caregivers will be called upon to play an even greater role in the care of the elderly, chronically ill patients and people with disabilities. Their expertise in basic care, their proximity to patients and their ability to build trusting relationships will be major assets in meeting these needs.

The rise of technology and the transformation of the business

Technological advances are revolutionizing the healthcare landscape. Telemedicine, connected objects, artificial intelligence and mobile applications are changing the way patients are cared for and monitored. For nursing assistants, this means adapting to new tools and increasing their digital skills. They will be required to use remote monitoring devices, collect and interpret health data, and collaborate via digital platforms. This technological transformation offers the opportunity to optimize care, increase efficiency and strengthen coordination with other healthcare professionals.

The importance of ongoing training

In view of these developments, ongoing training is becoming essential. Caregivers will need to regularly update their knowledge, acquire new skills and open up to emerging fields. Training will cover not only technical and technological aspects, but also patient-centered approaches, intercultural communication, stress management and ethics. Healthcare establishments and training organizations will have a key role to play in offering adapted, accessible and innovative programs.

Towards greater recognition of the profession

Enhancing the role of caregivers is a major challenge for the future. Recognition of their skills, expertise and essential contribution to the healthcare system must be reflected in career development prospects, adequate remuneration and full integration into care teams. Healthcare policies must support this recognition, by promoting professional development, encouraging access to training leading to qualifications, and raising the profile of the profession.

Innovation for people

Despite the rise of technology, the human aspect will remain at the heart of the nursing profession. Supporting patients as a whole, taking into account their physical, psychological, social and spiritual needs, remains a fundamental mission. Caregivers will continue to provide that irreplaceable human dimension of presence, listening, empathy and respect. Innovation must be seen as a tool in the service of this humanity, freeing up time for meaningful interaction and making care more personalized.

The challenges of diversity and inclusion

Society is becoming increasingly diverse, with populations from a variety of cultural, linguistic and religious backgrounds. Caregivers will need to develop intercultural communication skills, adapting their practices to respect the values and beliefs of each individual. This diversity is a source of richness, but it calls for heightened sensitivity and specific training to ensure fair and respectful care for all patients.

Prevention and health promotion

The future of healthcare is not limited to the treatment of disease, but also encompasses prevention and the promotion of well-being. Caregivers will have a greater role in health education, raising awareness of favorable behaviors, participating in prevention programs and encouraging self-management of chronic diseases. They will become key players in building a healthier society, collaborating with communities and getting involved in local initiatives.

Enhanced inter-professional collaboration

Teamwork will be more essential than ever. The boundaries between healthcare professions are tending to blur in favor of a collaborative, patient-centered approach. Caregivers will work closely with nurses, doctors, pharmacists, psychologists and social workers, sharing information, coordinating care and participating in clinical decisions. This interdisciplinary approach will enrich practices and improve the quality of care.

Ethical and regulatory challenges

Technological and societal developments also raise ethical and legal issues. The protection of personal data, informed consent, respect for privacy and fair access to care are all concerns that need to be taken into account. Caregivers will need to be trained in these issues, participate in ethical reflection and apply deontological principles in their daily practice.

The importance of professional well-being

To ensure quality care, it is essential to look after the well-being of the caregivers themselves. The profession is physically and emotionally demanding. The risks of burn-out, stress and musculoskeletal disorders are real. Healthcare establishments will need to implement prevention policies, promote a healthy working environment, offer psychological support and encourage work-life balance. Caregivers, for their part, will need to adopt self-care strategies, develop resilience and seek support when needed.

- Useful resources and references

To practise competently and stay up to date in a constantly evolving field like internal medicine, the nursing auxiliary needs to rely on reliable, up-to-date resources. This chapter offers a selection of essential references to guide your practice, enrich your knowledge and support your professional development. These resources cover various aspects of the profession, from fundamental textbooks to online platforms, professional organizations and continuing education.

Reference works and practical manuals

1. **"Guide de l'aide-soignant"** by Jean Chiariny and Anne-Marie Chiariny This book is a classic in the field, offering a comprehensive overview of the skills required, care techniques and theoretical knowledge needed for daily practice. It covers the practical aspects of the profession, fundamental care and patient communication, and includes updates on new recommendations.

2. **"Nursing in Medicine and Surgery"** by Brunner and Suddarth Although originally intended for nurses, this manual is a valuable resource for nursing assistants wishing to deepen their knowledge of medical pathologies and technical care. It offers a detailed understanding of diseases, treatments and associated nursing interventions.

3. **"Human Anatomy and Physiology"** by Elaine N. Marieb An essential work for mastering the basics of anatomy and physiology, enabling a better understanding

of how the human body functions and the mechanisms of pathologies encountered in Internal Medicine.

Professional organizations and associations

1. **Association Nationale des Aides-Soignants (ANAS)** ANAS represents nurses' aides at national level, offering professional support, information on legislative developments and continuing education opportunities. The ANAS website offers resources, news and discussion forums for exchanges with colleagues.

2. **International Council of Nurses (ICN)** Although focused on nurses, ICN provides resources relevant to caregivers, including best practices, ethics and professional development on an international scale.

Guidelines, protocols and regulations

1. **Your facility's care protocols** Each healthcare facility has its own specific protocols adapted to its practices. It is vital to consult them regularly to ensure that internal procedures for care, hygiene and safety are respected.

2. **Haute Autorité de Santé (HAS)** The HAS publishes good practice recommendations, methodological guides and opinions on the organization of care. These documents are essential for keeping abreast of national standards in healthcare quality and safety.

3. **Ministry of Solidarity and Health** The Ministry's official website provides information on health policies, current legislation, decrees relating to the nursing profession, and public health measures.

Continuing education and professional development

1. **Institut de Formation des Aides-Soignants (IFAS)** The IFAS offer initial and continuing training, specialization modules and practical workshops. They are a key resource for developing skills and updating knowledge.

2. **Agence Nationale du DPC (Développement Professionnel Continu)** The ANDPC offers accredited training programs, enabling caregivers to meet their continuing education obligations while improving their professional practices.

3. **Online training**

   - **MOOC Santé**: Online courses open to all, covering a variety of topics relevant to caregivers, such as palliative care, pain management, or communicating with patients.
   - **Specialized platforms**: Websites like "Formasup Santé" or "Espace Compétences" offer online training modules tailored to healthcare professionals.

Websites and online platforms

1. **Santé.fr** Official portal offering reliable information on diseases, treatments, healthcare facilities and medical news.

2. **Infirmiers.com** Although primarily aimed at nurses, this site offers articles, forums, educational resources and news that may be useful to nursing assistants.

3. **Online Medical Library** Access to scientific articles, medical journals and other resources to help you learn more about specific topics.

Trade magazines and newspapers

1. **"Soins Aides-Soignantes"** This professional magazine features articles on care practices, feedback, thematic dossiers and information on developments in the profession.

2. **"Revue de l'Infirmière"** Although focused on the nursing profession, this publication offers interesting perspectives on nursing practices, healthcare innovations and current issues in the sector.

3. **"Le Concours médical"** Generalist magazine covering many aspects of medicine, useful for keeping up to date with scientific advances and ethical debates.

Useful mobile applications

1. **Medscape** Application offering medical news, drug information, clinical guides and useful calculation tools for healthcare professionals.

2. **Measuring vital signs** Apps like "iCare Health Monitor" can measure certain vital signs (heart rate, oxygen saturation) using sensors integrated into smartphones, useful for quick checks (use with caution and do not replace approved medical devices).

3. **Urgence santé** Application providing emergency protocols, first aid procedures and useful numbers, practical for reviewing emergency gestures.

Literature on personal and professional development

1. **"Emotional Intelligence"** by Daniel Goleman This book explores the importance of emotional skills in

interpersonal relationships, a key aspect for caregivers in supporting patients.

2. **"Prendre soin de soi pour prendre soin des autres"** by Philippe Rodet This book offers thoughts and advice on how to manage stress, prevent burnout and maintain a healthy work-life balance.

Support organizations and programs

1. **Occupational health services** These services offer support to prevent occupational hazards, propose workstation adjustments if necessary, and support caregivers in their well-being at work.

2. **Psychological support associations** Organizations such as the Association Soins aux Professionnels de Santé (SPS) offer psychological support to caregivers facing difficulties, stress or burn-out.

Ethics and deontology resources

1. **Comité Consultatif National d'Éthique (CCNE)** The CCNE publishes opinions and reports on health-related ethical issues, offering in-depth reflections on complex subjects encountered in healthcare practice.

2. **Codes of ethics** Although caregivers do not have a specific code of ethics, referring to the codes of the medical and paramedical professions can provide important ethical benchmarks.